theclinics.com

HAND CLINICS

Humerus Fractures

GUEST EDITOR
Scott P. Steinmann, MD

November 2007 • Volume 23 • Number 4

SAUNDERS
An Imprint of Elsevier, Inc.
PHILADELPHIA LONDON TORONTO MONTREAL SYDNEY TOKYO

W.B. SAUNDERS COMPANY
A Division of Elsevier Inc.

1600 John F. Kennedy Blvd. • Suite 1800 • Philadelphia, Pennsylvania 19103

http://www.theclinics.com

HAND CLINICS
November 2007
Editor: Debora Dellapena

Volume 23, Number 4
ISSN 0749-0712
ISBN-13: 978-1-4160-5077-3
ISBN-10: 1-4160-5077-9

Hand Clinics (ISSN 0749-0712) is published quarterly by Elsevier Inc., 360 Park Avenue South, New York, NY 10010-1710. Months of publication are February, May, August, and November. Business and Editorial Offices: 1600 John F. Kennedy Blvd., Suite 1800, Philadelphia, PA 19103-2899. Customer Service Office: 6277 Sea Harbor Drive, Orlando, FL 32887-4800. Periodicals postage paid at New York, NY, and additional mailing offices. Subscription price is $261.00 per year (U.S. individuals), $454.00 per year (U.S. institutions), $133.00 per year (US students), $297.00 per year (Canadian individuals), $454.00 per year (Canadian institutions), $164.00 (Canadian students), $333.00 per year (international individuals), $454.00 per year (international institutions), and $164.00 per year (international students). Foreign air speed delivery is included in all *Clinics* subscription prices. All prices are subject to change without notice. POSTMASTER: Send address changes to *Hand Clinics*, Elsevier Periodicals Customer Service, 6277 Sea Harbor Drive, Orlando, FL 32887-4800. **Customer Service: 1-800-654-2452 (US). From outside the US, call 1-407-345-4000. E-mail: hhspcs@harcourt.com.**

Reprints. For copies of 100 or more, of articles in this publication, please contact the Commercial Rights Department, Elsevier Inc., 360 Park Avenue South, New York, NY 10010-1710. Tel: (212) 633-3813, Fax: (212) 462-1935, e-mail: reprints@elsevier.com.

Hand Clinics is covered in *Index Medicus, Current Contents/Clinical Medicine, EMBASE/Excerpta Medica,* and *ISI/BIOMED.*

Printed in the United States of America.

GUEST EDITOR

SCOTT P. STEINMANN, MD, Associate Professor of Orthopedic Surgery, Department of Orthopedic Surgery, Mayo Clinic, Rochester, Minnesota

CONTRIBUTORS

WAYNE Z. BURKHEAD, MD, Shoulder and Elbow Service, The Carrell Clinic, Dallas, Texas

EMILIE V. CHEUNG, MD, Assistant Professor, Department of Orthopedic Surgery, Stanford University, Stanford, California

PETER A. COLE, MD, Chief of Orthopaedic Surgery, Regions Hospital; Professor, Division of Orthopaedic Trauma, Department of Orthopaedic Surgery, University of Minnesota, Saint Paul, Minnesota

CHARLES M. COURT-BROWN, MD, FRCSEd(Orth), Professor of Orthopaedic Trauma, Royal Infirmary of Edinburgh, Edinburgh, Scotland

ANNA R. KING, BA, Department of Orthopedic Surgery, Mayo Clinic, Rochester, Minnesota

SUMANT G. KRISHNAN, MD, Shoulder and Elbow Service, The Carrell Clinic, Dallas, Texas

MARGARET M. McQUEEN, MD, FRCSEd(Orth), Consultant Orthopaedic Surgeon, Royal Infirmary of Edinburgh, Edinburgh, Scotland

STEVEN L. MORAN, MD, Associate Professor of Plastic Surgery, Department of Plastic Surgery, Mayo Clinic, Rochester, Minnesota

JOHN R. REINECK, MD, Shoulder and Elbow Service, The Carrell Clinic, Dallas, Texas

DAVID RING, MD, PhD, Hand and Upper Extremity Service, Partners Orthopaedic Trauma Service, Department of Orthopaedic Surgery, Massachusetts General Hospital, Boston, Massachusetts

M. WADE SHRADER, MD, Vice-Chairman, The CORE Institute, Phoenix, Arizona

SCOTT P. STEINMANN, MD, Associate Professor of Orthopedic Surgery, Department of Orthopedic Surgery, Mayo Clinic, Rochester, Minnesota

THOMAS W. THROCKMORTON, MD, Department of Orthopedic Surgery, Mayo Clinic, Rochester, Minnesota

GILLES WALCH, MD, Centre Orthopédique Santy, Lyon, France

BRYAN WALL, MD, The CORE Institute, Phoenix, Arizona

COEN A. WIJDICKS, MSc, Research Fellow, Department of Orthopaedic Surgery, University of Minnesota, Minneapolis, Minnesota

PETER C. ZARKADAS, MD, Department of Orthopedic Surgery, Mayo Clinic, Rochester, Minnesota

CONTENTS

FORTHCOMING ISSUES

February 2008

Acute and Chronic Elbow Instability
Scott G. Edwards, MD, *Guest Editor*

May 2008

Contemporary Issues Related to Management of the Upper Limb in Tetraplegia
Albert A. Weiss, MD, and
Mary Jane Mulcahey, PhD, OTR/L,
Guest Editors

August 2008

Thumb Arthritis
Tamara D. Rozental, MD, *Guest Editor*

RECENT ISSUES

August 2007

The Ulnar Nerve
Dan A. Zlotolow, MD, and
Vincent D. Pellegrini, Jr, MD, *Guest Editors*

May 2007

Forearm Injuries
Marco Rizzo, MD, *Guest Editor*

February 2007

Microsurgical Reconstruction of the Upper Extremity: State of the Art
Neil F. Jones, MD, *Guest Editor*

ELSEVIER
SAUNDERS

Hand Clin 23 (2007) ix

HAND
CLINICS

Preface

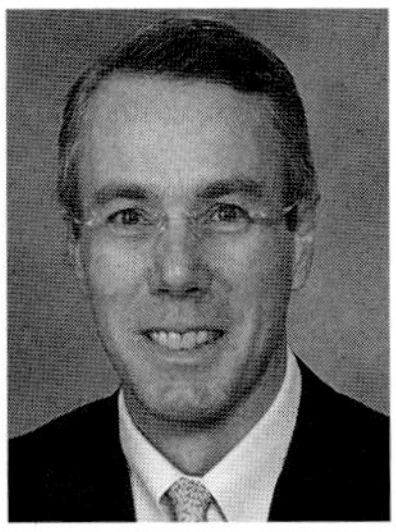

Scott P. Steinmann, MD
Guest Editor

This issue of *Hand Clinics* is devoted to the treatment of humerus fractures. Recent changes in the incidence and treatment of these fractures are important to highlight. There has been an increase in the incidence of fractures, both in elderly osteoportic patients and in the young mobile patient. Unique challenges exist in addressing osteoporotic bone and in providing solutions for the young active patient.

In the past, humerus fractures, both proximal and distal, were treated nonoperatively, and it was expected that they would "all do well." This was recommended due to both a lack of technology and a lack of reliable studies of treatment outcomes. Much has changed in the last two decades; biomechanical studies and clinical studies have availed us of new techniques and procedures.

Proximal humerus fractures are now treated with several methods, including plating, pinning, and even reverse total shoulder replacement. Midshaft humerus fractures, which a generation ago were treated mainly with nonoperative means are being stabilized with different operative techniques. Distal humerus fractures, which as a resident I felt were the most difficult fractures to treat in either the upper or lower extremity, now have several surgical treatment options. No longer is "bag-of-bones" treatment thought of as a viable treatment in the active individual. Lastly, articular fractures of the humerus are better understood as the convergence of greater imaging technology, specific internal fixation advancements, and postoperative treatments have combined to yield better patient outcomes.

I would like to thank all the authors of this issue who were asked to contribute due to their known expertise on humerus trauma. Also, this issue could not have been done without the guidance of Debora Dellapena.

Scott P. Steinmann, MD
Department of Orthopedic Surgery
Mayo Clinic
200 First Street, SW
Rochester, MN 55902, USA

E-mail address: Steinmann.Scott@mayo.edu

doi:10.1016/j.hcl.2007.09.005

hand.theclinics.com

ELSEVIER
SAUNDERS

Hand Clin 23 (2007) 397–414

HAND
CLINICS

Two-Part Fractures and Fracture Dislocations

Charles M. Court-Brown, MD, FRCSEd(Orth)*,
Margaret M. McQueen, MD, FRCSEd(Orth)

Royal Infirmary of Edinburgh, Old Dalkeith Road, Edinburgh EH16 4SU, Scotland

Proximal humeral fractures are common, with a recent epidemiologic analysis estimating the incidence at 63/100,000 per year [1], and they are osteopenic or osteoporotic. A recent prospective study of 1027 proximal humeral fractures from Edinburgh, Scotland, showed an average patient age of 66, with the highest age-specific prevalence being in women between 80 and 89 [2]. The study showed that 73% of proximal humeral fractures occurred in women with an average age of 70 and 27% occurred in men with an average age of 56.

Two commonly used classification and outcome systems are used. The classifications are those of Neer [3] and the Orthopaedic Trauma Association (OTA), the latter being derived from the AO classification [4]. The outcome studies are those of Neer [3] and Constant [5] although, as with other fractures, several outcome systems exist, which increases the complexity of interpreting the literature. Fortunately, however, many of the recent articles examining the treatment of proximal humeral fractures use either the Neer or the Constant scores and, where possible, both are used in this article to facilitate comparison with other studies in the literature.

Neer [3] described four two-part fractures and two two-part fracture dislocations. The two-part fractures were defined as fractures of the anatomic neck, surgical neck, greater tuberosity, and lesser tuberosity in which displacement was more than 1 cm or the angulation between the fragments was more than 45°. The two-part fracture dislocations involved a fracture of the tuberosities and were either anterior or posterior in direction. Neer's classification relies on a definition of displacement that is often difficult to apply in the clinical situation. In virtually all articles in the literature, the displacement has been measured from nonstandardized radiographs and considerable error is involved in the process. In addition, the Neer classification does not include all the different types of two-part surgical neck fractures that are encountered by surgeons.

The OTA classification is morphologic and makes no allowance for displacement. It is based on the location of the fracture, the presence of impaction, angulation, translation or comminution of the surgical neck, and the presence or absence of a dislocation. Neer's two-part fractures are OTA type A fractures, with the greater tuberosity fractures and fracture dislocations being A1 fractures, and the six types of surgical neck fractures being A2 and A3 fractures (Fig. 1). The A2.1 fracture is a fracture of the surgical neck that is undisplaced in the coronal plane but displaced in the sagittal plane. The A2.2 fracture is a varus-impacted fracture and the A2.3 fracture is a valgus-impacted fracture. In the A3 group, the fractures are unimpacted, with the A3.1 fracture being an angulated fracture and the A3.2 fracture a translated fracture. The A3.3 fracture has metaphyseal comminution.

Neer's and Constant's outcome criteria measure objective and subjective factors in assessing the patient's final outcome. The ability to carry out activities of daily living is analyzed, as is shoulder function and mobility. Constant also developed a graph of normal shoulder function (Fig. 2), which shows the diminution of shoulder function with increasing age, important when

* Corresponding author.
E-mail address: courtbrown@aol.com (C.M. Court-Brown).

doi:10.1016/j.hcl.2007.08.003

hand.theclinics.com

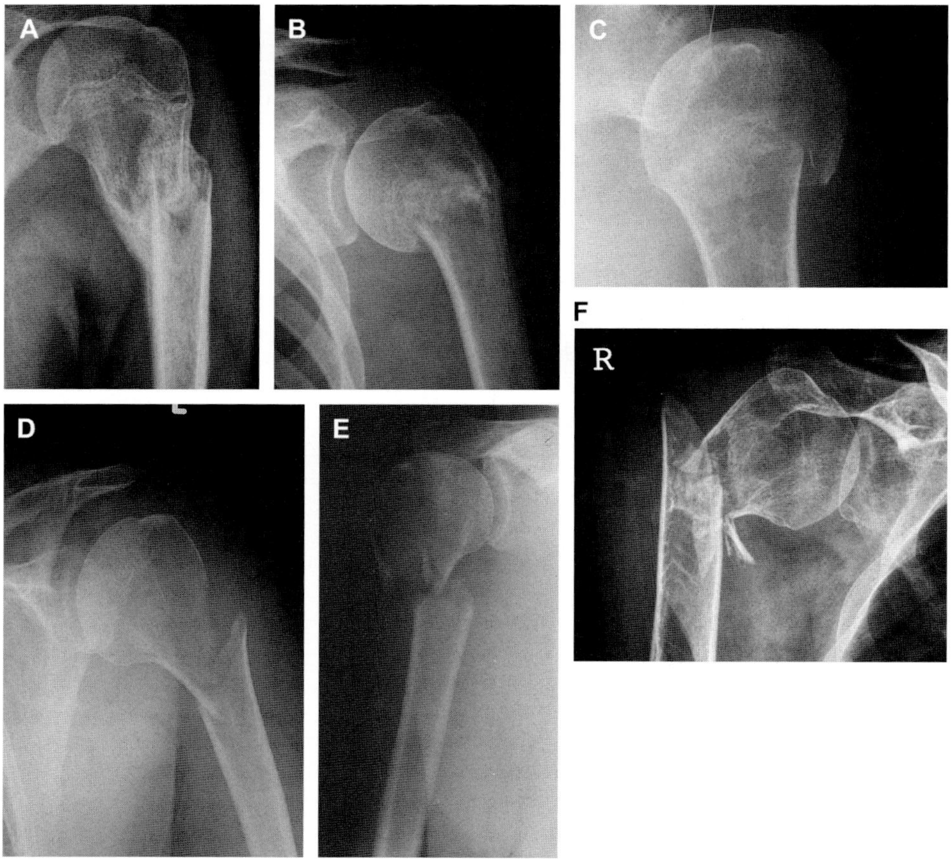

Fig. 1. OTA A2 and A3 surgical neck fractures. (*A*) A2.1 fracture. It has united, but shows the displacement in the sagittal plane. (*B*) A2.2 impacted varus fracture. (*C*) A2.3 impacted valgus fracture. (*D*) A3.1 angulated fracture. (*E*) A3.2 translated fracture. (*F*) A3.3 fracture showing metaphyseal comminution.

analyzing the literature. Initially, a raw Constant score is calculated that takes no account of the patient's age, but an age-corrected Constant score can be calculated by comparing the affected shoulder with the normal shoulder. In this article, raw Constant scores have been used where possible. It is important to know whether the raw Constant or the age-corrected Constant score is being used. Soete and colleagues [6], in their article on Kirschner wiring (K-wiring) of proximal humeral fractures, used both Constant scores, and showed that if the raw Constant score was used, they had 38% excellent and good results, but if the corrected Constant score was used, they had 81% excellent and good results. This discrepancy can obviously lead to confusion.

This article adheres to Neer's basic definition of two-part fractures but subclassifies them according to the OTA classification. The epidemiology and nonoperative management section is based on the prospective database collected by Court-Brown and colleagues [2] over a 4-year period in Edinburgh, Scotland. The authors have published articles on the two most common variants of the surgical neck fracture, the A3.2 translated fracture [7] and the A2.2 impacted varus fracture [8], but, because these articles were based on the OTA classification, they included minimally displaced fractures according to Neer's definition. In this article, only two-part fractures are considered.

One other drawback about combining Neer's displacement criteria with the OTA classification is that some type B and C fractures are two-part fractures because only one of the fractures in the proximal humerus is displaced sufficiently to satisfy Neer's criteria. This scenario occurred in 47 of the 1027 fractures analyzed by Court-Brown and colleagues and was mainly seen in the common

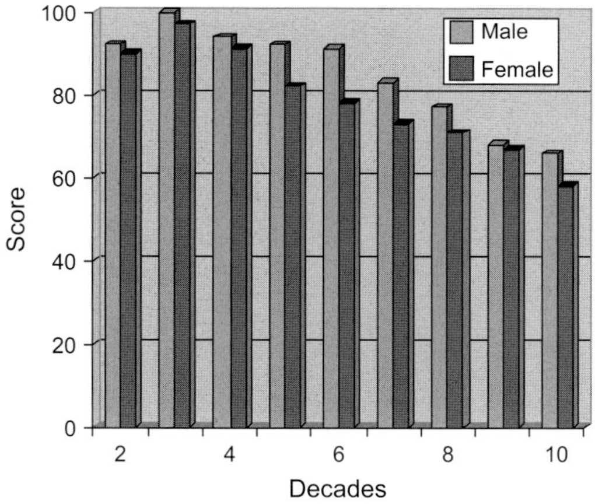

Fig. 2. Correlation of age and Constant score. Note the marked deterioration in normal shoulder function after about 60 years of age. (*From* Constant CR. Age related recovery of shoulder after injury [thesis]. Cork (Ireland): University College Cork; 1986; with permission.)

impacted bifocal B1.1 fracture, where either the greater tuberosity or the surgical neck was significantly displaced. These fractures have not been included in the analysis contained in this article.

Epidemiology

The epidemiology of proximal humeral fractures is changing. Horak and Nilsson [9] estimated that 4% of fractures involved the proximal humerus, whereas about 30 years later, Court-Brown and Caesar [1] found that 5.7% of fractures involved the proximal humerus. In 1970, Neer [3] stated that 85% of proximal humeral fractures were minimally displaced, whereas in 2001, Court-Brown and colleagues [2] found that 49% of proximal humeral fractures were minimally displaced. The differences are accounted for by increasing longevity and osteoporosis in the population. Osteoporotic fractures tend to be more comminuted and displaced, and therefore, the prevalence of displaced proximal humeral fractures in the population has increased, compared with a generation ago. Table 1 shows the epidemiology of two-part fractures and fracture dislocations taken from Court-Brown and McQueen's prospective study. The 287 displaced two-part fractures and fracture dislocations indicated a prevalence of 27.9% of all proximal humeral fractures. Only 15% of fractures occurred in patients younger than 50, and 30% occurred in patients older than 80. More than two thirds of the fractures occurred in women. The importance of separating the different types of surgical neck fractures is also highlighted in Table 1. The A2 fractures, which include the impacted A2.2 and A2.3 fractures, occur in older patients, whereas the unimpacted A3 fractures tend to have a slightly lower average age. The angulated A3.1 fracture and the A3.3 fracture associated with metaphyseal comminution occur in the

Table 1
Epidemiology of Neer two-part fractures taken from the study of Court-Brown and McQueen

Fracture type	N	M/F (%)	Average age (y)	<50 y (%)	≥80 y (%)
Surgical neck fractures	232	24/76	70	12	34
A2.1 (sagittal malalignment)	7	71/29	71	14	43
A2.2 (varus impaction)	51	16/84	73	2	29
A2.3 (valgus impaction)	18	11/89	78	0	56
A3.1 (unimpacted, angulated)	14	65/35	51	43	29
A3.2 (unimpacted, translated)	120	24/76	72	11	38
A3.3 (metaphyseal comminution)	22	50/50	61	32	9
Greater tuberosity fractures	10	50/50	66	30	30
A1.2	10	50/50	66	30	30
Fracture dislocations					
A1.3	45	47/53	58	33	13
Anterior	43	49/51	58	33	14
Posterior	2	0/100	54	50	0
Total	287	31/69	67	15	30

The Neer two-part fractures have been subclassified using the OTA (AO) classification.

youngest groups of patients. The most common two-part fracture is the A3.2 translated surgical neck fracture, and about 40% of these occur in patients older than 80, a fact that is of considerable importance when considering management.

Displaced A1.2 two-part greater tuberosity fractures are surprisingly few. In fact, the Court-Brown and colleagues series had 148 greater tuberosity fractures [2], but 46 were completely undisplaced and 92 were considered to be displaced by less than 1 cm. Table 1 shows that the 10 displaced fractures occurred equally in men and women, with an average age of 66. Of the 45 two-part fracture dislocations, only 2 were posterior, the remaining 43 being anterior. The average age of the fracture dislocation group was lower than that of the proximal humeral fracture group. The average age of the A1.2 minimally displaced greater tuberosity fracture group was 56, indicating that, as patients age, the fractures tend to be more severe.

Treatment

Much has been written about the treatment of two-part proximal humeral fractures, but with remarkably little agreement about the optimal method, and, given the frequency with which surgeons encounter these fractures, it is surprising how few large studies of their management have been undertaken. Several studies have concentrated on younger patients and in many studies two-, three-, and four-part fractures have been combined, so it is difficult to analyze the results. Many of the articles dealing with proximal humeral fractures come from level 1 trauma centers or specialized shoulder centers, which deal mostly with the complications of proximal humeral fractures rather than with a large number of fresh fractures. Thus, the implication is that most proximal fractures are handled surgically, but the authors believe that, given the age of the patients who present with these fractures, most are probably, in fact, treated nonoperatively in the community. Despite this, little information about the results of nonoperative management has existed until recently. The authors present the Edinburgh results of the use of nonoperative management in all type A fractures and fracture dislocations. They do not seek to tell surgeons that all fractures should be treated nonoperatively, but the information may be helpful when comparing the results of different treatment methods.

Nonoperative treatment

In the two-part fractures and fracture dislocations listed in Table 1, eight greater tuberosity fractures, 200 surgical neck fractures, and 36 greater tuberosity anterior fracture dislocations were treated nonoperatively apart from reduction of the dislocation. One of the posterior fracture dislocations was treated nonoperatively. The overall results for the two-part greater tuberosity fractures, surgical neck fractures, and anterior fracture dislocations are presented in Table 2. The 1-year Neer and Constant scores are similar, although the best results of nonoperative management occurred in the A3.1 group, where, at 1 year, the average Neer score was 90 and the average raw Constant score was 76. Table 1, however, indicates that this fracture occurred in a younger group of patients with an average age of 51. The worst results occurred in the A2.3 impacted valgus group and the A3.3 group with metaphyseal comminution. Both groups had an average Neer score of less than 80 after 1 year. The A2.3 group was the oldest, with an average age of 78 and, although the average age of the A3.3 group was 61, evidence now indicates that metaphyseal comminution leads to nonunion and this group had two nonunions. Patients in the A3.3 group also tended to have more medical and social comorbidities, which may explain the low scores.

A2.1 fractures

A2.1 fractures are relatively common. Court-Brown and colleagues' prospective study had 98 [2], although only 7 were two-part fractures. The rest were minimally displaced, and at 1 year, the minimally displaced A2.1 group had an average Neer score of 85 and an average Constant score of 69. Table 2 shows that the seven two-part A2.1 fractures also did well with nonoperative management and at 1 year had an average Neer score of 84 and an average Constant score of 64.

A2.2 impacted varus fractures

Table 2 shows that the average Neer and Constant scores were 83 and 66, respectively, at 1 year. A review of the Constant graph correlating shoulder function with age (see Fig. 1) indicates that in a population with an average age of 73, these results are good. In a previous study, Court-Brown and McQueen [8] analyzed the results of treating 99 A2.2 fractures, although 48 of these were minimally displaced. Some orthopedic surgeons are concerned that the varus impaction associated

Table 2
The outcome scores for all two-part fractures and two-part fracture dislocations treated nonoperatively

	Outcome scores (1 year)			Neer's outcome criteria (1 year)		
Type	N	Neer	Constant	Excellent	Satisfactory	Total[a]
Surgical neck[b]						
A2	76	82	64	32.7	36.7	69.4
A2.1	7	84	64	20.0	80.0	100.0
A2.2	51	83	66	28.9	42.1	71.0
A2.3	18	78	59	45.4	18.2	63.6
A3	124	81	65	40.0	25.4	65.4
A3.1	10	90	76	50.0	50.0	100.0
A3.2	95	81	64	39.6	27.1	66.7
A3.3	19	76	63	25.0	12.5	37.5
A2 and A3	200	81	65	36.1	30.6	66.7
Greater tuberosity						
A1.2	8	86	74	33.3	50.0	83.3
Dislocations						
A1.3	35	84	71	45.1	29.0	74.1

The numbers of fractures treated nonoperatively are shown.
[a] The sum of the excellent and satisfactory results.
[b] The surgical neck section includes results for the different OTA fracture subgroups, for the A2 and A3 groups, and for all surgical neck fractures (A2 and A3 combined).

with an A2.2 fracture will lead to impingement between the greater tuberosity and the acromion, resulting in pain. All 99 patients were nonoperatively managed and the overall Neer score at 1 year was 87, indicating that the minimally displaced fractures fared slightly better than the two-part fractures. Analysis of the varus angle showed no statistical correlation between age and the initial varus angle but age and the final varus angle were correlated, indicating an association between increasing osteopenia and an increasing varus angle. However, final varus angle and outcome were not statistically correlated, with patients who had a varus angle of 40° to 49° at 1 year still having an average Neer score of 84. An increasing varus angle and pain were also not correlated, indicating that symptomatic acromial impingement was not a problem. Analysis of the Neer score at 1 year showed that the patient's subjective score of stability, reach, and strength were about 90% of normal, whereas flexion averaged 70% of the normal arm and abduction only 53% of normal. Flexion and abduction power were about 70% of normal.

Analysis of the 99 A2.2 fractures with relation to age showed that increasing age was associated with a poorer result and greater impairment of shoulder function. Age correlated with the overall Neer score and with decreasing reach, flexion abduction, and internal rotation, and, in fact, was the main predictor of outcome. However, age and pain were not statistically correlated. A review of the two-part A2.2 fractures (Table 3) indicates that the older age groups have decreased function, although patients over 80 still have an average Neer and Constant score of 78 and 61, respectively, at 1 year.

A3.2 translated fracture

The A3.2 translated fracture is the commonest two-part surgical neck fracture and has received the most attention in the literature. Nonoperatively managed A3.2 fractures have average Neer and Constant scores of 81 and 64, respectively, at 1 year (see Table 2) and, given the average age of 72, these scores compare well with the Constant age outcome graph (see Fig. 1). Table 3 shows an association between outcome and increasing age.

In 2001, Court-Brown and colleagues [7] examined the management of the translated two-part fracture in detail. They excluded five physeal fractures, and showed that, as with the A2.2 fracture, age and the Neer score were statistically correlated at 1 year. The return of flexion and abduction in older patients was particularly poor. The investigators also examined the association

Table 3
Effect of increasing age on the outcomes of nonoperatively treated proximal humeral fractures and dislocations

	≤50 y		51–60 y		61–70 y		71–80 y		>80 y	
Fracture	N	C	N	C	N	C	N	C	N	C
A2.2	—	—	84	69	85	70	83	65	78	61
A3.2	94	78	96	83	87	76	80	61	70	50
A1.3	96	90	88	75	70	52	78	61	81	64
	<65 y		≥65 y							
	N	C	N	C						
A2.3	75	57	80	59						
A3.1	92	73	87	72						
A3.3	77	66	74	58						
A1.2	91	85	83	66						

Where the number of fractures was less than 20, data were insufficient to subdivide the scores into decades, and the data have been presented above and below 65 years of age. No good data for A2.1 fractures existed because only two patients were younger than 75. Data for patients younger than 50 who had A2.2 fractures were also not worthwhile.

Abbreviations: C, Constant score; N, Neer score.

between outcome and increasing surgical neck translation. They showed that increasing translation of the humeral head on the proximal shaft correlated with increasing age. The patients who presented with up to 33% translation had an average age of 73, whereas the patients who had more than 100% translation had an average age of 78. The degree of translation also correlated with function at 1 year, with the group with translation of up to 33% having a Neer score of 85, compared with 67 for the older group with complete translation. They also compared operative and nonoperative management in the patients with more than 66% translation and found virtually identical Neer scores at 1 year in both groups, although the operative group was significantly younger than the nonoperative group.

Little information exists about nonoperative management elsewhere in the literature, although Fjalestad and colleagues [10] examined a group of 13 A3 fractures, 5 of which were treated nonoperatively and 8 of which were treated operatively. They used a different outcome measure, but could find no evidence that surgical intervention in A3 fractures improved their results. Kristiansen and Christensen [11] analyzed 26 surgical neck fractures treated nonoperatively or by plate fixation and reviewed the patients at an average of 4 years after injury. The median Neer scores showed no significant difference between the two groups. Olsson and colleagues [12] reviewed four nonoperatively managed surgical neck fractures 13 years after injury and found an average Constant score of 59. They drew attention to the substantial mortality in patients who had proximal humeral fractures and found that displacement and medical comorbidities were associated with poorer results.

A2.3 impacted valgus fractures

No studies have been undertaken on the A2.3 surgical neck fracture. Table 1 shows that it has the highest average patient age and the authors' series had only one patient under 70, which presumably explains the apparent lack of correlation between age and outcome shown in Table 3. All patients were treated nonoperatively, with average 1-year Neer and Constant scores of 78 and 59, respectively (see Table 2). The authors believe that the lower scores reflect the higher age of this group.

A3.1 angulated fractures

No previous studies of this fracture have been done. The authors treated 26 fractures in a 4-year period, of which 14 were two-part fractures. Five patients were younger than 20, which accounts for the low average age of the group (see Table 1). The Neer and Constant scores for the nonoperatively managed two-part fractures were 90 and 76, respectively (see Table 2), which indicates a good result. Four patients were treated surgically, but their average age was 17. Their Neer and Constant scores at 1 year were 90 and 80, respectively, suggesting that nonoperative management works well. The average Neer and Constant scores at 1 year for the minimally displaced A3.1 fractures were 90 and 78, respectively, indicating that in this fracture, initial displacement does not indicate a worse prognosis.

A3.3 fractures with metaphyseal comminution

No previous studies of this fracture have been done. The authors treated 46 patients in 4 years, but 24 were minimally displaced fractures. In the 19 that were treated nonoperatively, the average Neer and Constant scores at 1 year were 76 and 63, respectively (see Table 2), which represents the poorest functional result of any surgical neck fracture. The results of the minimally displaced A3.3 group at 1 year were 86 and 70, respectively. As with other fractures, the results of the A3.3 nonoperatively managed group deteriorated with advancing age (see Table 3). It is likely that the relatively poorer results seen in the A3.3 fractures are caused by the metaphyseal comminution associated with nonunion and to the number of medical comorbidities in this group. Two of the A3.3 fractures failed to unite and both had a poor functional outcome. Nonunion is discussed further in the section relating to complications.

Plate fixation

Conventional plating methods

The literature regarding the use of conventional plates in proximal humeral fractures (Fig. 3) has concentrated mainly on the management of three- and four-part fractures. Investigators have often combined the results of the treatment of two-, three-, and four-part fractures, and it is often difficult to tease out the results of two-part fractures. Table 4 shows the results of seven articles dealing with the use of conventional plates. Most surgeons have used a T-plate inserted through a deltopectoral approach and have used Neer's outcome criteria. Few indications have been given for operative treatment except for displacement, and generally, surgeons do not comment on age as an indication for surgery.

Paavolainen and colleagues [13] treated 20 displaced surgical neck fractures but, as is frequently the case with this elderly group of patients, they were only able to follow up 15 patients. However, they reported 14 excellent or satisfactory results. The results of Kristiansen and Christensen [14] were not as good. They treated six surgical neck fractures and reported on five; the sixth patient developed deep infection. Their complication rate was high, with infection in three cases, implant loosening in one case, and implant malposition in one case. Moda and colleagues [15] reported on a very small number of patients, but all six patients who had surgical neck fractures had excellent or satisfactory results. However, the average age was between 20 and 40, and was not representative of most populations who sustain two-part fractures.

Robinson and Christie [16] not only undertook a comparative study of plate fixation versus intramedullary fixation with Rush nails but examined the effect of age on their results. The overall average Neer score for 22 patients who had two-part

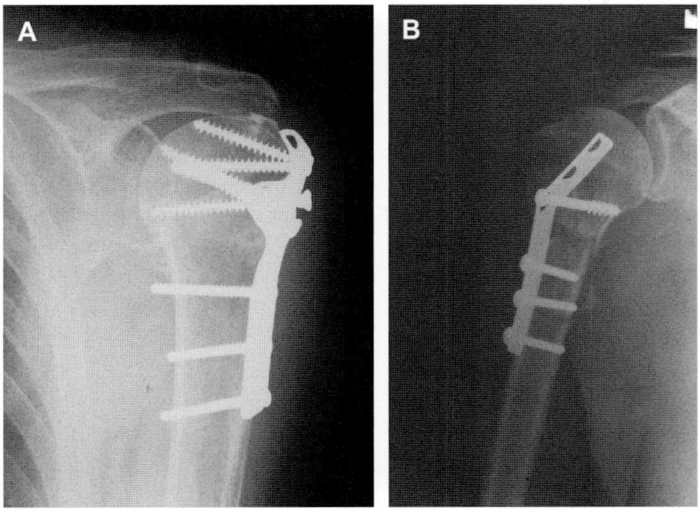

Fig. 3. Examples of conventional plate fixation. (*A*) A lateral plate. Note it is slightly high and there is evidence of screw loosening. (*B*) A bent one-third tubular plate used to treat the fracture shown in Fig. 1E. It is used as a blade plate.

Table 4
Results from the literature of the use of conventional plating techniques in Neer two-part surgical neck fractures

	N	Fracture type	Age[a] (y)	Neer criteria: Neer score	Neer criteria: Excellent/Satisfactory (%)	Constant score	Plate type
Paavolainen, et al [13]	15	A2:A3	61	89	93	—	T
Kristiansen and Christensen [14]	5	A2:A3	53	76	—	—	T
Moda, et al[b] [15]	6	A2:A3	20–40	—	100	—	Blade
Robinson and Christie [16]	22	A2:A3	—	76	41	—	T
	8		<50	89	88	—	T
	14		>60	51	14	—	T
Szyszkowitz, et al[c] [17]	42	A2:A3	—	—	65	—	T (55%)
Hessmann, et al [18]	50	A2:A3	—	—	62	—	T
Wanner, et al [19]	10	A2:A3	62	—	—	67	One-third tubular
Total/averages	150	—	60	81	64	67	—

[a] Average ages are given unless specified otherwise.
[b] The "blade" plate used by Moda et al was a bent one-third tubular plate.
[c] The study by Szyszkowitz et al used a number of different implants but 55% were T-plates. The average Neer and Constant scores are given.

surgical neck fractures treated with a T-plate was 76, but it rose to 89 if the patient was younger than 50. In the over-60 group, only 2 of 14 patients had an excellent or satisfactory outcome. They noted a high incidence of implant failure in this group that was usually attributed to loosening of the screws in the humeral head. No Rush pins were used in patients younger than 50, but in the older group, 69% had excellent or satisfactory results following the use of Rush pins.

Szyszkowitz and colleagues [17] treated 42 two-part surgical neck fractures but used various techniques, although 55% of the patients were treated with T-plates. In this study, 89.7% of proximal humeral fractures were treated nonoperatively and the investigators stated that A2 and A3 fractures might require surgery if closed reduction failed. They reported 65% excellent and satisfactory results using Neer's criteria, but the age of the patient group was not specified.

Hessmann and colleagues [18] had very similar results, with 62% excellent and satisfactory results using Neer's criteria. They attributed their poor results to fracture malreduction and injury to the rotator cuff. A particular problem was varus deformity of more than 15° that led to a restricted range of shoulder movement. Both Paavolainen and colleagues [13] and Hessmann and colleagues [18] stressed the importance of not applying the T-plate too high on the humeral head and thereby causing impingement. Wanner and colleagues [19] used a different technique. They used two one-third tubular plates and a deltopectoral approach. They treated 10 two-part surgical neck fractures and reported only one complication of plate breakage, although the patient apparently did well. The average Constant score was 67 in a population with an average age of 62, which compares well with nonoperative management (see Table 2).

Complications of conventional plating relate mainly to the age of the patient. Most authorities agree that the principal problem is screw failure in the humeral head, leading to varus malposition. This problem is closely related to osteoporosis and is a greater problem in older patients. Other problems include subacromial impingement from a high plate, plate breakage, and nonunion (see later discussion). Infection is relatively uncommon, varying from 0% to 12.5% in the studies in Table 4. It is usually impossible to separate septic arthritis in two-part fractures from septic arthritis in three- and four-part fractures, and if the total number of proximal humeral fractures in the articles listed in Table 4 is considered, the 455 patients had 11 infections, giving a prevalence of 2.4%.

Locking plates

The problems associated with the use of conventional plates in the treatment of proximal humeral fractures have encouraged surgeons to use locking plates, where the screws engage with the plate and the bone (Fig. 4). The theory is that screw failure will not occur, secondary varus malalignment will be minimized, and the results will be better. Because the implants are relatively new, the literature is still deficient. Several articles have not provided functional results and outcome has been assessed radiologically and by the prevalence of complications. Another problem is that by the time these articles were written the Constant score had become more popular, but some articles do not indicate whether they are using the raw or the age-adjusted Constant score. However, available results are summarized in Table 5. As with conventional plates, locking plates are usually inserted through an anterior deltopectoral incision, although in recent years, more surgeons have been using deltoid splitting approaches.

Saudan and colleagues [20] treated eight surgical neck fractures and reported good results, although their results were clearly better in younger patients. They had relatively minor complications, as did Koukakis and colleagues [22] (2006). However, other investigators have reported a higher incidence of complications. Babst and colleagues [23] treated 111 patients, including 61 two-part surgical neck fractures. They reported that 16 screws perforated the humeral head and 12 (10.8%) patients had a secondary loss of reduction. No infections were reported. Rose and colleagues [24] also had a relatively high complication rate. They treated 16 patients, including four two-part fractures, and reported a high prevalence of nonunion (25%), which they attributed to metaphyseal comminution, smoking, and medical comorbidities. They also theorized that diaphyseal extension may not be well treated by conventional locking plates. Agudelo and colleagues [25] reported on the use of locking plates in four level 1 trauma centers in the United States and Germany. The study included 147 fractures, of which 19% were type A fractures. They reported that 14% of the fractures had screw cut out, loss of reduction, or plate failure and that, as with conventional plating, varus malreduction and delayed mechanical failure were related. They also reported 4.8% infection. Similar results were reported by Owsley and Gorczyca [26] in 75 proximal humeral fractures, of which 20 were type A fractures. Sixty-nine were treated with angular stable plates, but overall varus collapse occurred in 20% of cases. Smith and colleagues [27] had no varus collapse in 22 patients treated with locking plates, but 27.3% of patients showed delayed healing and 18.2% required secondary surgery.

Bjorkenheim and colleagues [28] analyzed 32 patients who had two-part surgical neck fractures and reported better results. The average Constant score for these patients was 84 after one year compared with 78 and 60 for the three and four-part

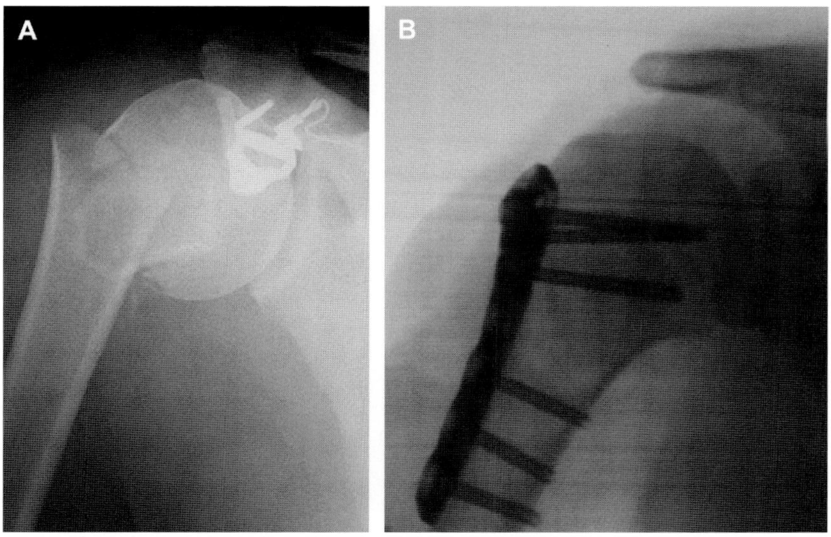

Fig. 4. Angular stable locking plate. (*A*) A high energy displaced surgical neck fracture in a 34-year-old man. (*B*) A locked plate has been used. Good reduction was achieved.

Table 5
Results from the literature of the use of angular stable locked Philos plates

	N	Fracture type	Age (y)	Constant score	Plate type
Saudan, et al [20]	8	A3	64	60[a]	Philos
	—	—	<65	73	—
	—	—	≥65	52	—
Björkenheim, et al [28]	32	A2:A3	67	84	Philos
Fankhauser, et al [21]	4	A3	64	83	Philos
Koukakis, et al [22]	3	A2:A3	58	88	Philos
Kettler, et al [29]	61	A2:A3	66	67	Philos
Babst, et al [23]	61	A2:A3	64	76	Philos
Total/averages	169	—	65	74	—

[a] The results of Saudan et al comprise a mixture of two- , three-, and four-part fractures.

fractures. They combined their fractures and showed that outcome related to age. The average Constant score for patients younger than 50 was 85, but was 59 for those patients older than 80. They reported very few complications.

The studies reported in Table 5 have all used the Philos plate, but other fixed angle locking plates have been used. The PlantTan plate has been examined by several groups of surgeons, but its use has been discontinued by two groups because of screw penetration through the humeral head [30] and an unacceptably high infection rate together with fixation failure [31].

The findings in Table 5 point to improved results, when compared with conventional plating and with nonoperative management, although Table 5 represents only one plate manufactured by one company. Given the apparent problems associated with the use of the PlantTan plate [30,31], more work is clearly required on the role of locking plates in these fractures. Different opinions are expressed in the literature, and Frangen and colleagues [32] expressed a view that, in more complex fractures, angular stable implants did not show improved functional outcome when compared with alternative fixation devices. It is also clear that varus malposition and screw penetration of the glenohumeral joint do occur. However, it would seem that these plates represent an advance, although this seeming advance may be due to early optimism; more work must be done to compare their use with other treatment methods and to analyze their use in different age groups.

Intramedullary nailing

As with plating, much of the clinical research investigating the use of intramedullary nailing in proximal humeral fractures has been in three- and four-part fractures, but several studies have been undertaken examining their use in two-part fractures or in mixed groups of proximal humeral fractures. Intramedullary nailing of proximal humeral fractures takes two forms. Some surgeons favor antegrade nailing, using either a long nail adapted from a humeral diaphyseal nail or short nails specifically designed for the proximal humerus. Other surgeons have used retrograde pinning, a technique derived from the earlier Hackethal pinning technique [33]. The theoretic advantage of nailing over plating is that much less dissection is required, but the obvious potential disadvantage of antegrade nailing is rotator cuff damage, particularly in this older group of patients. In theory, retrograde pinning should combine minimal dissection with cuff integrity but, outside mainland Europe, the technique has not become popular.

Antegrade nailing

Robinson and Christie [16] examined the use of Rush nails inserted through the greater tuberosity and supplemented by a tension band around the greater tuberosity (Fig. 5). They stressed the importance of meticulous cuff repair and, using Neer's outcome criteria, they reported 76% excellent and good results in older patients (Table 6). However, the technique was not problem free, and, out of 23 patients, they reported 12 secondary operative procedures, with 9 patients requiring Rush pin removal because of shoulder discomfort. They reported four fixation failures and two wound infections, although no deep infections occurred.

Lin and colleagues [34] reported on the use of antegrade nailing (see Fig. 5) in 21 two-part surgical neck fractures. They used a long humeral nail with proximal screws that could be passed

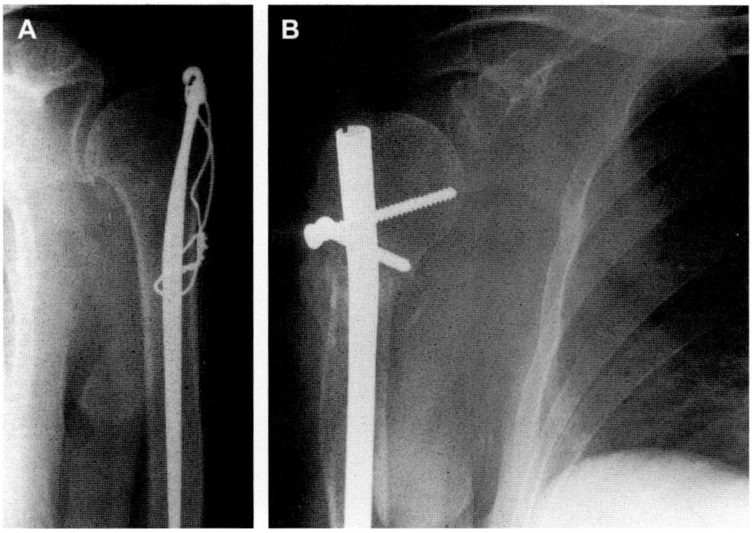

Fig. 5. Examples of antegrade intramedullary nailing. (*A*) The use of Rush pins and a tension band. Note the prominence of the pins and the potential for rotator cuff damage. (*B*) A conventional, dynamically locked antegrade intramedullary nail.

upwards into the humeral head or downwards into the metaphysis. Table 6 shows that they reported more excellent and satisfactory results than Robinson and Christie [16], but it seems likely that the average age of the patient group was lower. They reported no deep infections, implant failure, osteonecrosis, or nail migration, but it is obvious from the article that some patients had significant proximal protrusion of the nail.

In recent years, the use of the Polaris nail has been examined by several surgeons. Rajasekhar and colleagues [35] documented its use in 23 two-part fractures. They reported similar results to other surgeons and that better results occurred in younger patients (see Table 6). They reported one nonunion and one case of severe shoulder stiffness, but no infection, implant failure, malunion, or nail migration.

Linhart and colleagues [36] reported on the use of the Targon nail, which is essentially a Polaris nail with more proximal screw holes. They treated 25 two-part surgical neck fractures and reported an average Constant score of 64. Functional

Table 6
Results from the literature of the use of antegrade intramedullary nailing in Neer two-part surgical neck fractures

	n	Fracture type	Age[a] (y)	Neer score	Excellent/ Satisfactory (%)	Constant score	Nail type
Robinson and Christie [16]	21	A2:A3	>60	84	76 (N)	—	Rush pins
Lin, et al [34]	21	A2:A3	66	87	86 (N)	—	No name
Rajasekhar et al [35]	23	A2:A3	65	—	80 (C)	—	Polaris
			≤60	—	85	—	
			>60	—	75	—	
Linhart, et al [36]	25	A2:A3	72	—	—	64	Targon
Total/averages	90	—	68	85	73 (N) 80 (C)	64	—

Neer and Constant outcome measures were used in these studies and average excellent and satisfactory scores are given for both scoring systems.

Abbreviations: C, Constant score; N, Neer score.

[a] Average ages are given unless specified otherwise.

outcome improved up to 1 year but not after this time. As reported in most other articles, they found deteriorating shoulder function with increasing age. They reported few complications in their two-part fracture group, with minor problems of screw loosening only. No infections occurred.

Analysis of Table 6 shows that the overall Neer and Constant scores for antegrade intramedullary nailing of two-part surgical neck fractures are virtually the same as for nonoperative management (see Table 2) and conventional plating (see Table 4), although the average age of the patients is much closer to the average age of the patients treated by nonoperative management. The average Constant score for antegrade intramedullary nailing is less than that of locked plating with a similar average age. Overall, antegrade intramedullary nailing appears to have no advantage over nonoperative management or conventional plating, probably not surprising given the age of the patient group being treated and the inevitable rotator cuff damage associated with the technique. Antegrade nailing for humeral diaphyseal fractures has been abandoned by many surgeons because of shoulder dysfunction secondary to rotator cuff damage. It will be surprising if this is not the case in proximal humeral fracture patients who are, on average, 10 years older than patients who have humeral diaphyseal fractures.

Retrograde pinning

The use of retrograde pins to stabilize proximal humeral fractures was popularized by Hackethal [33]. It is a closed technique, with pins or flexible nails being inserted distally and advanced proximally to stabilize the reduced proximal humeral fracture. The pins are usually inserted in the distal humerus above the elbow, but shorter pins or wires can be inserted in the proximal humeral diaphysis. In recent years, the Helix spring and the J nail have been so inserted.

The overall results for retrograde pinning are shown in Table 7. Zifko and colleagues [37], Qidwai [38], and Habernek and colleagues [39] have all published the results of retrograde pinning with a distal humeral entry point. Qidwai [38] used K-wires, but his population was so different from the average population of proximal humeral fractures that his results are probably going to be difficult to emulate. The average age of his patient group was 28, and he actually excluded elderly patients. Clearly, the technique seems to work in this unusual group of patients.

The other articles listed in Table 7 have a more conventional patient population. Zifko and colleagues [37] reported about 58% excellent and satisfactory results using Neer's criteria, but Habernek and colleagues [39] had better results, with an average Neer score of 80. This article is virtually unique in that it subdivides two-part

Table 7
Results from the literature of the use of retrograde intramedullary pinning in Neer two-part surgical neck fractures

	n	Fracture type	Age[a] (y)	Neer score	Excellent/ Satisfactory (%)	Constant score	Pin type
Zifko, et al [37]	25	A2:A3	60		58[b] (N)	—	Zitter
Habernek, et al [39]	26	A3	63	80	—	—	Spiral bundle
	5	A3.1	67	84	—	—	
	15	A3.2	61	76	—	—	
	6	A3.3	65	85	—	—	
Qidwai [38]	18	A2:A3	28	—	100 (N)	—	K-wires
Takeuchi, et al [42]	40	A2:A3	65	88	90[b] (N)	—	J nail
Raissadat, et al [41]	4	A2:A3	77	—	—	68	Helix
Gorschewsky, et al [40]	32	A2:A3	70	—	69[b] (C)	95[c]	Helix
Total/averages	145	—	61	84	84 (N) 69 (C)	68	—

Neer and Constant outcome measures were used in these studies and average excellent and satisfactory scores are given for both scoring systems.

Abbreviations: C, Constant score; N, Neer score.

[a] Average age.

[b] Results include non–two-part proximal humeral fractures.

[c] Gorschewsky et al used the age-adjusted Constant score.

fractures and presents the results of retrograde pinning in A3.1, A3.2, and A3.3 fractures. The results are shown in Table 7. Note the contrast with nonoperative management (see Table 2). The A3.1 angulated fracture and the A3.2 translated fracture appear to do better if managed nonoperatively, but retrograde nailing of A3.3 fractures with metaphyseal comminution seems to give better results. Habernek and colleagues [39] did not report nonunion in the A3.3 fracture group, which other investigators have done, and this omission may be relevant when comparing the different results.

The complications of the technique are relatively few, although Qidwai [38] and Habernek and colleagues [39] reported six cases of elbow stiffness (33% and 23%, respectively). Zifko and colleagues [37] reported seven cases, giving an overall prevalence of 30% in the three studies. The other problem is humeral head penetration by the pins for the same reasons as in locked plating. In osteopenic or osteoporotic patients, the proximal humerus impacts downwards and the pins and screws may penetrate the head.

The alternative method of inserting retrograde pins or wires through the proximal humeral diaphysis is less popular. The usefulness of the titanium Helix spring has generated considerable controversy, with Gorschewsky and colleagues [40] publishing 68.5% very good and good results using Constant's outcome criteria. A contrary view is taken by Raissadat and colleagues [41], who treated nine two-part fractures, but only published results on four fractures. However, in their combined 15 two- and three-part fractures, they had 7 (47.6%) nonunions and they recommended that the Helix device not be used.

The use of the J nail was investigated by Takeuchi and colleagues [42]. The J nail is, in fact, a K-wire with the proximal end bent into a J-shape. Three wires are passed from just below the deltoid muscle insertion, across the reduced proximal humeral fracture. The investigators reported a good result in a group of patients with an average age of 65. They reported that older patients had poorer results, although they still had an average Neer score of 83 in patients aged 80.

Too little good information exists to make a judgment on the usefulness of these nails. In theory, retrograde shoulder pinning could prove to be effective because of the minimal dissection, but more studies must be undertaken before their use can be recommended. The results shown in Table 7 are very similar to those of nonoperative management and conventional plating.

Kirschner wires

Several surgeons have used percutaneously inserted K-wires to stabilize proximal humeral fractures (Fig. 6). As with other methods of fixation, these have been mainly used in three- and four-part fractures, but several investigators have reported their use in two-part surgical neck fractures. Kocialkowski and Wallace [43] treated 18 two-part surgical neck fractures but they only had good results in patients younger than 50. In this group, they had 100% excellent results, according to Neer's outcome criteria. Only 19% of patients older than 50 had excellent or satisfactory results. They reported 23% pin track sepsis and 41% K-wire migration, with one pin entering the chest wall. One radial nerve palsy was reported.

Chen and colleagues [44] analyzed the use of percutaneous screws or pins in two- and three-part proximal humeral fractures. They reported results of nine surgical neck fractures, but the average age was 35.4 and three patients were younger than 15. The average Neer score was 94, and 89% had excellent or satisfactory results. They reported no

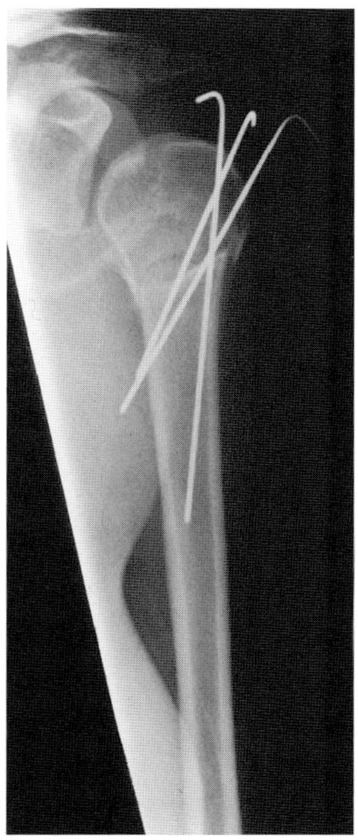

Fig. 6. Use of K-wires to treat a surgical neck fracture in a young man.

infections and only two cases of pin migration. Herscovici and colleagues [45] reported on the use of K-wires and threaded wires in 21 two-part surgical neck fractures. The average age of the patient group was 49; about 50% of patients were injured in motor vehicle accidents; and the study included one open two-part fracture. They used different outcome criteria and reported good results with threaded pins, but not with unthreaded K-wires. The results of isolated fractures were better than those in multiply injured patients.

In a recent study, Keener and colleagues [46] treated seven surgical neck fractures in patients with an average age of 70. They reported good results, with a final mean Constant score of 79. The found no difference in results according to age, but they reported two varus deformities and one pin loosening. The results in this study are good, but only seven patients were studied. All other articles have essentially reported good results in younger patients and the authors would concur with the view that this technique is much less successful in older osteoporotic bone.

External fixation

Periarticular external fixation has been used for two-part proximal humeral fractures, although the technique is not in widespread use. Kristiansen and Kofoed [47] treated 31 displaced proximal humeral fractures by external fixation and nonoperative management. Most of the fractures were three- and four-part fractures, but they treated four two-part fractures by external fixation and three nonoperatively. Two of their three nonoperatively managed patients developed nonunion and had poor results. Unfortunately, they did not separate the results for their externally fixed two-, three-, and four-part fractures, but the median Neer score was 79, and 73% had excellent or satisfactory results, according to Neer's criteria.

In a more recent study, Martin and colleagues [48] used periarticular external fixation in 40 two-part fractures and 22 three-part fractures. The patients had a mean age of 70. The overall mean age–corrected Constant score was 84, and complications were few. Given the age of the patients, these results appear good, but more studies are required to identify the place of external fixation.

Other methods

Surgeons have used sutures and wire loops to reconstruct the proximal humerus, but these techniques are mostly used in three- and four-part fractures and in greater tuberosity fractures. However, Cornell and colleagues [49] used a tension band passed under the supraspinatus proximally and through the lateral cortex distally to treat eight two-part surgical neck fractures. It was reported that 10 of 13 patients who had two- and three-part fractures had a good result.

Complications

Because most proximal humeral fractures occur in elderly patients, several complications can be expected. The authors have already outlined the technical complications associated with the different treatment methods, but, in a recent study, Hoxie and colleagues [50] quoted 5.1% pulmonary embolus in 137 consecutive patients treated surgically. In a study from the same institution, Smith and colleagues [27] examined 82 shoulders that had had osteosynthesis and showed that 51.2% had a nonmedical complication, 25.6% required secondary surgery, and 2.4% developed deep infection.

The problem of nonunion (Fig. 7) is often discussed, and it has been stated that nonunion

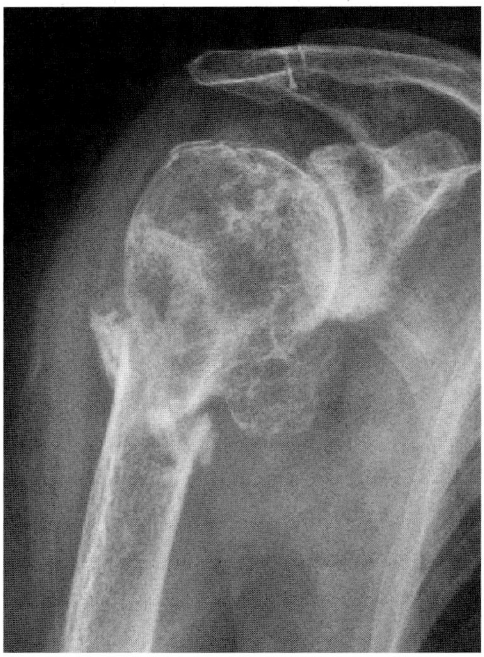

Fig. 7. Proximal humeral nonunion. This fracture was an A3.3 fracture in a middle-aged alcoholic man.

occurs in about 20% of proximal humeral fractures and is associated with nonoperative management [51]. This finding is patently incorrect because no fracture occurring in cancellous bone has such a high nonunion rate. In their consecutive series of 1027 fractures, Court-Brown and McQueen [2] had 11 (1%) nonunions. In a recent study of these nonunions [52], they showed that six occurred in two-part surgical neck fractures, giving a prevalence of 2.1%. The study reported no nonunions in greater tuberosity fractures. The highest rate in two-part fractures was in A3.2 fractures, with 4.3% nonunions; increased translation was associated with a higher rate of nonunion, although, paradoxically, the group with complete displacement of the surgical neck had no nonunions. Two A3.3 and two B2.3 fractures, associated with metaphyseal comminution, developed nonunion, meaning that 7.7% of all fractures with metaphyseal comminution developed nonunion. Court-Brown and McQueen [52] showed that age was also a factor, but nonoperative management was not.

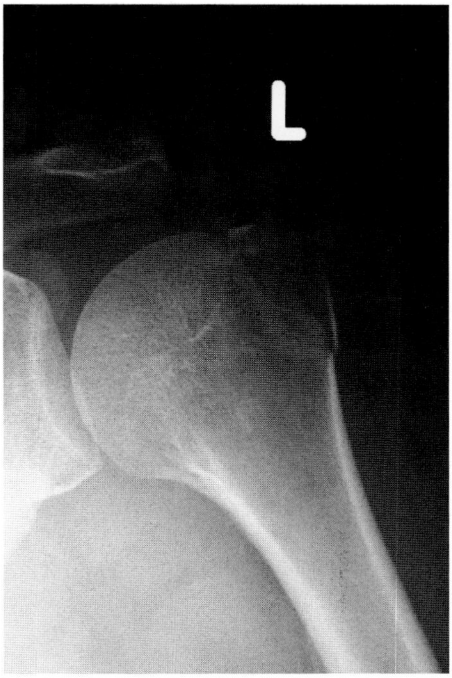

Fig. 8. A1.2 greater tuberosity fracture. This fracture has displaced posteriorly, and accurate measurement of the displacement is not possible.

Greater tuberosity fractures

In the series of 1027 proximal humeral fractures reported by Court-Brown and McQueen [2], 102 (10%) were A1.2 greater tuberosity fractures (Fig. 8), but only 10 were displaced by more than 1 cm (see Table 1). The average age was 66, compared with 56 for the minimally displaced A1.2 fractures. Table 2 shows that the results of nonoperative management were good and Table 3 shows a definite relationship with increasing age.

The permissible degree of displacement of the greater tuberosity is being debated. Many surgeons will fix the tuberosity if displacement is greater than 5 mm, although others will accept up to 1 cm. Little evidence supports either view. Platzer and colleagues [53] examined shoulder function in 125 patients who had minimally displaced greater tuberosity fractures. They sought to measure 1- to 5-mm greater tuberosity displacement in nonstandardized radiographs and they showed that the Constant score associated with 1-mm displacement was 83, compared with 75 for 5-mm displacement. The results were not statistically different. The Constant score for the authors' nonoperatively managed group with about 10-mm displacement was virtually identical (see Table 2). These results suggest that there are two important factors to consider. First, nonstandardized radiographs are virtually impossible to measure accurately and second, it is rare for the greater tuberosity fragment to be displaced by much more than 1 cm without significant rotator cuff damage. It seems likely that nonoperative management of most A1.2 fractures will give good results, but marked displacement means cuff damage, requiring surgery.

Lesser tuberosity fractures

Lesser tuberosity fractures are very rare but may have been associated with a posterior fracture subluxation. Most are treated nonoperatively, unless displacement is significant.

Anatomic neck fractures

Anatomic neck fractures are also rare. The Court-Brown and McQueen series [2] had no two-part unimpacted OTA C1.3 fractures, which is the classic Neer two-part anatomic neck fracture. However, the series did have three two-part type C fractures (C1.1, C2.2, and C2.3), with an average patient age of 61. Treatment depends on displacement and patient age. Fractures may be nonoperative, or displaced fractures may be treated by internal fixation in younger patients and by hemiarthroplasty in older patients.

Surgical neck fracture dislocations

Surgical neck fracture dislocations are rare and probably occur mainly in debilitated osteoporotic patients. An example is shown in Fig. 9. Treatment is by open reduction and internal fixation.

Greater tuberosity fracture dislocations

Anterior

Table 1 shows that these tend to occur in younger patients, and that age has a major effect on outcome (see Table 3). The mechanism of the tuberosity fracture is debated, with some surgeons suggesting that the fracture is an avulsion fracture and others that it is an impaction fracture from contact with the glenoid or acromion during dislocation [54]. The authors believe that two types of fracture dislocation exist. Type I is an avulsion fracture, with the bone fragment being pulled off by the rotator cuff (see Fig. 9). This fracture is associated with considerable displacement. Type II is a presumed impaction fracture associated with less displacement (see Fig. 9). Type I fractures should be treated as cuff avulsions, and, if the patient is fit, repair is indicated, although, because these patients are usually elderly, the outcome is sometimes uncertain. The treatment of type II fractures is essentially that of the displaced A1.2 fracture, although an ultrasound or MRI examination of the integrity of the cuff should be undertaken in older patients. Table 2 shows that 35 patients who had two-part fracture dislocations managed nonoperatively did very well but the results are age dependent (see Table 3). Over a decade, Dimakopoulos and colleagues [55] surgically treated 36 patients who had A1.3 fracture dislocations. The average age was 53 and the average Constant score was 88. They did not record their indications or whether they operated on every patient.

Posterior

Two-part posterior fracture dislocations are rare. They tend to occur in younger patients (see Table 1) but little is known about their outcome. If more information is required, the review by Robinson and Aderinto [56] should be consulted.

Suggested treatment

The authors believe that the data presented in this article suggest that, at the moment, nonoperative is the "default" position in the

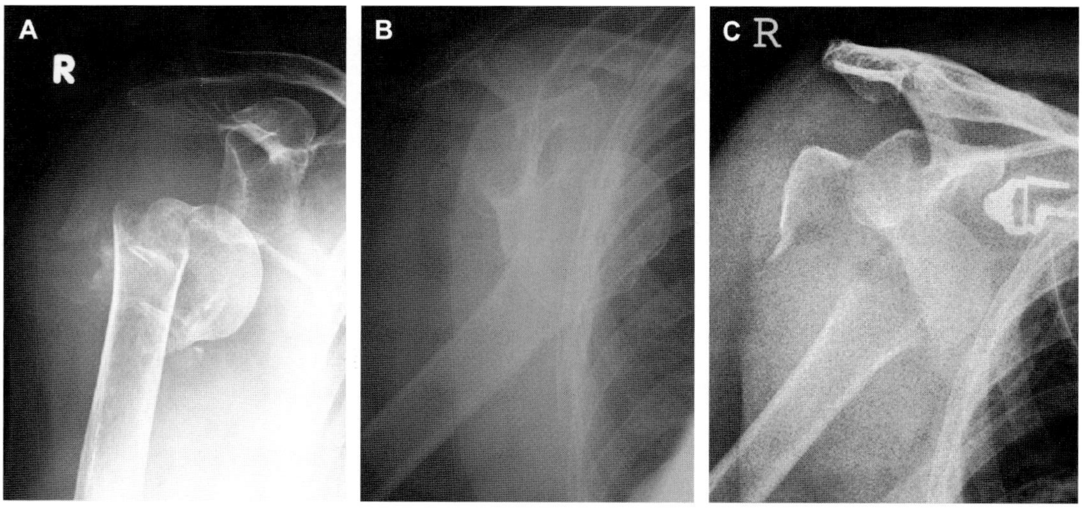

Fig. 9. The three types of anterior fracture dislocation. (*A*) A surgical neck fracture dislocation. These fractures are very rare and little is known about the results of their management. (*B*) A type I A1.3 greater tuberosity fracture dislocation. This avulsion fracture of the greater tuberosity is associated with considerable rotator cuff damage. (*C*) A type II impingement greater tuberosity fracture dislocation, which is usually associated with less damage to the rotator cuff.

treatment of two-part surgical neck fractures! Evidence is good that the results of conventional plating, antegrade nailing, and K-wiring are no better in older patients. The results of all fixation techniques are good in younger patients, but these patients are not the problem. Locked plating seems to give good results and may well be a useful technique, but one must balance understandable initial enthusiasm with proven success. Comparative studies between locked plating and nonoperative management in the elderly are required. Retrograde pinning seems reasonably successful, but the results are not much better than those of nonoperative management.

It is likely that surgical techniques will improve, but patients are getting older and frailer. Studies are required to prove the benefits of surgery in a rapidly aging population.

References

[1] Court-Brown CM, Caesar B. The epidemiology of adult fractures. Injury 2006;37:691–7.

[2] Court-Brown CM, Garg A, McQueen MM. The epidemiology of proximal humeral fractures. Acta Orthop Scand 2001;72:365–71.

[3] Neer CS. Displaced proximal humeral fractures. Part 1. Classification and evaluation. J Bone Joint Surg Am 1970;52:1077–89.

[4] Müller ME, Nazarian S, Koch P, et al. The comprehensive classification of fractures of long bones. New York: Springer-Verlag; 1990.

[5] Constant CR. Age related recovery of shoulder function after injury [thesis]. University College Cork; 1986.

[6] Soete PJ, Clayson PE, Costenoble VH. Transitory percutaneous pinning in fractures of the proximal humerus. J Shoulder Elbow Surg 1999;8:569–73.

[7] Court-Brown CM, Garg A, McQueen MM. The translated two-part fracture of the proximal humerus: epidemiology and outcome in the older patient. J Bone Joint Surg Br 2001;83:799–804.

[8] Court-Brown CM, McQueen MM. The impacted varus (A2.2) proximal humeral fracture. Acta Orthop Scand 2004;75:736–40.

[9] Horak J, Nilsson BE. Epidemiology of fracture of the upper end of the humerus. Clin Orthop Relat Res 1975;112:250–3.

[10] Fjalestad TY, Strømsøe K, Blücher J, et al. Fractures in the proximal humerus: functional outcome and evaluation of 70 patients treated in hospital. Arch Orthop Trauma Surg 2005;125:310–6.

[11] Kristiansen B, Christensen SW. Proximal humeral fractures. Acta Orthop Scand 1987;58:124–7.

[12] Olsson C, Nordquist A, Petersson CJ. Long-term outcome of a proximal humerus fracture predicted after 1 year. Acta Orthop 2005;76:397–402.

[13] Paavolainen P, Björkenheim J-M, Slätis P, et al. Operative treatment of severe proximal humeral fractures. Acta Orthop Scand 1983;54:374–9.

[14] Kristiansen B, Christensen SW. Plate fixation of proximal humeral fractures. Acta Orthop Scand 1986;57:320–3.

[15] Moda SK, Chadha NS, Sangwan SS, et al. Open reduction and fixation of proximal humeral fractures and fracture-dislocations. J Bone Joint Surg Br 1990;72:1050–2.

[16] Robinson CM, Christie J. The two-part proximal humeral fracture: a review of operative treatment using two techniques. Injury 1993;24:123–5.

[17] Szyszkowitz R, Seggl W, Schleifer P, et al. Proximal humeral fractures: management and expected results. Clin Orthop Relat Res 1993;292:13–25.

[18] Hessmann M, Baumgaertel F, Gehling H, et al. Plate fixation of proximal humeral fractures with indirect reduction: surgical technique and results utilizing three shoulder scores. Injury 1999;30:453–62.

[19] Wanner GA, Wanner-Schmid E, Hersche O, et al. Internal fixation of displaced proximal humeral fractures with two one-third tubular plates. J Trauma 2003;54:536–44.

[20] Saudan M, Stern RE, Lubbeke A, et al. Fixation of fractures of the proximal humerus: experience with a new locking plate. In: Program and abstracts of the Orthopaedic Trauma Association; 2003.

[21] Fankhauser F, Boldin C, Schippinger G, et al. A new locking plate for unstable fractures of the proximal humerus. Clin Orthop Relat Res 2005;430:176–81.

[22] Koukakis A, Apostolou CD, Taneja T, et al. Fixation of proximal humerus fractures using the PHILOS plate: early experience. Clin Orthop Relat Res 2006;442:115–20.

[23] Babst RH, Sommer C, Bahrs C, et al. Open reduction and internal fixation (ORIF) of proximal humeral fractures with an angular stable form plate: an international multicenter analysis of outcome and complications. In: Program and abstracts of the Orthopaedic Trauma Association; 2006.

[24] Rose PS, Adams CR, Torchia ME, et al. Locking plate fixation for proximal humeral fractures: initial results with a new implant. J Shoulder Elbow Surg 2007;16:202–7.

[25] Agudelo JF, Schürmann M, Stahel PF, et al. Analysis of efficacy and failure in proximal humeral fractures treated with angular stable locking plates. In: Program and abstracts of the Orthopaedic Trauma Association; 2005.

[26] Owsley KC, Gorczyca JT. Fracture displacement and hardware migration after open reduction and internal fixation of proximal humeral fractures. In: Program and abstracts of the Orthopaedic Trauma Association; 2006.

[27] Smith AM, Mardones RM, Sperling JW, et al. Early complications of operatively treated proximal humeral fractures. J Shoulder Elbow Surg 2007;16:14–24.

[28] Björkenheim J-M, Pajarinen J, Savolainen V. Internal fixation of proximal humeral fractures with a locking compression plate. Acta Orthop Scand 2004;75:741–5.

[29] Kettler M, Biberthaler P, Braunstein V, et al. Die winkelstabile osteosynthese am proximalen humerus mit der Philos-platte. Unfallchirurg 2006;109:1032–40.

[30] Sadowski C, Riand N, Stern R, et al. Fixation of fractures of the proximal humerus with the PlantTan humerus fixator plate: early experience with a new implant. J Shoulder Elbow Surg 2003;12:148–51.

[31] Machani B, Sinopidis C, Brownson P, et al. Mid term results of PlantTan plate in the treatment of proximal humeral fractures. Injury 2006;37:269–76.

[32] Frangen TN, Dudda M, Arens S, et al. Proximal humeral fractures with angle-stable plate osteosynthesis: is everything better now? In: Program and abstracts of the Orthopaedic Trauma Association; 2006.

[33] Hackethal KH. Die Bündel-Nagelung. Berlin: Springer; 1961.

[34] Lin J, Hou SM, Hang YS. Locked nailing for displaced surgical neck fractures of the humerus. J Trauma 1998;45:1051–7.

[35] Rajasekhar C, Ray PS, Bhamra MS. Fixation of proximal humeral fractures with the Polaris nail. J Shoulder Elbow Surg 2001;10:7–10.

[36] Linhart W, Ueblacker P, Großterlinden L, et al. Antegrade nailing of humeral head fractures with captured interlocking screws. J Orthop Trauma 2007;21:285–94.

[37] Zifko B, Poigenfürst J, Pezzei C, et al. Flexible intramedullary pins in the treatment of unstable proximal humeral fractures. Injury 1991;22:60–2.

[38] Qidwai SA. Treatment of proximal humeral fractures by intramedullary Kirschner wires. J Trauma 2001;50:1090–5.

[39] Habernek H, Schneider R, Popp R, et al. Spiral bundle nailing of subcapital humeral fractures: preliminary report of the method of Henning. J Trauma 1999;46:400–6.

[40] Gorschewsky O, Puetz A, Klakow A, et al. The treatment of proximal humeral fractures with intramedullary titanium helix wire by 97 patients. Arch Orthop Trauma Surg 2005;125:670–5.

[41] Raissadat K, Struben P-J, van Loon CJM. Helix wire osteosynthesis for proximal humeral fractures: unacceptable union rate in two- and three-part fractures. Arch Orthop Trauma Surg 2004;124:166–8.

[42] Takeuchi R, Koshino T, Nakazawa A, et al. Minimally invasive fixation for unstable two-part proximal humeral fractures: surgical techniques and clinical results using J-nails. J Orthop Trauma 2002;16:403–8.

[43] Kocialkowski A, Wallace WA. Closed percutaneous K-wire stabilization for displaced fractures of the surgical neck of the humerus. Injury 1990;21:209–12.

[44] Chen CY, Chao EK, Tu YK, et al. Closed management and percutaneous fixation of unstable proximal humerus fractures. J Trauma 1998;45:1039–45.

[45] Herscovici D, Saunders DT, Johnson MP, et al. Percutaneous fixation of proximal humeral fractures. Clin Orthop Relat Res 2000;375:97–104.

[46] Keener JD, Parsons BO, Flatow EL, et al. Outcomes after percutaneous reduction and fixation of proximal humeral fractures. J Shoulder Elbow Surg 2007;16:330–8.

[47] Kristiansen B, Kofoed H. Transcutaneous reduction and external fixation of displaced fractures of the proximal humerus. A controlled clinical trial. J Bone Joint Surg Br 1988;70:821–4.

[48] Martin C, Guillen M, Lopez G. Treatment of 2- and 3-part fractures of the proximal humerus using external fixation. Acta Orthop 2006;77:275–8.

[49] Cornell CN, Levine D, Pagnani MJ. Internal fixation of proximal humeral fractures using the screw-tension band technique. J Orthop Trauma 1994;8:23–7.

[50] Hoxie SC, Sperling JW, Cofield RH. Pulmonary embolism after operative treatment of proximal humeral fractures. J Shoulder Elbow Surg, in press.

[51] Warner JJ, Coustouros JG, Gerber C. Fractures of the proximal humerus. In: Bucholz RW, Heckman JD, Court-Brown C, editors. Rockwood and Green's fractures in adults. 6th edition. Philadelphia: Lippincott, Williams and Wilkins; 2006. p. 1161–210.

[52] Court-Brown CM, McQueen MM. Nonunions of the proximal humerus. Their prevalence and functional outcome. J Trauma, in press.

[53] Platzer P, Kutscha-Lissberg F, Lehr S, et al. The influence of displacement on shoulder function in patients with minimally displaced fractures of the greater tuberosity. Injury 2005;36:1185–9.

[54] Bahr C, Lingenfelter E, Fischer F, et al. Mechanism of injury and morphology of the greater tuberosity fracture. J Shoulder Elbow Surg 2006;15:140–7.

[55] Dimakopoulos P, Panagopolos A, Kasimatis G, et al. Anterior traumatic shoulder dislocation associated with displaced greater tuberosity fracture: the necessity of operative treatment. J Orthop Trauma 2007;21:104–12.

[56] Robinson CM, Aderinto J. Posterior shoulder dislocations and fracture-dislocations. J Bone Joint Surg Am 2005;87:639–50.

ELSEVIER
SAUNDERS

Hand Clin 23 (2007) 415–424

HAND
CLINICS

Four-Part Proximal Humerus Fractures: Evaluation and Treatment

John R. Reineck, MD, Sumant G. Krishnan, MD*, Wayne Z. Burkhead, MD

Shoulder and Elbow Service, The Carrell Clinic, 9301 North Central Expressway, Suite 400, Dallas, TX 75231, USA

Proximal humerus fractures represent 4% to 5% of all fractures and are the most common fractures of the shoulder girdle. Retrospective epidemiologic reviews have demonstrated that proximal humerus fractures accounted for 53% of all significant shoulder girdle injuries [1]. Most of these fractures are the result of a fall, and the female-to-male ratio is 2:1. Furthermore, increasing age has been shown to correlate with increasing fracture risk in women, suggesting an association with osteoporosis. Fractures of the humerus also represent the third most common fracture in the elderly (with only hip fractures and Colles' fractures being more common), and the prevalence of proximal humeral fractures in the elderly has been increasing in recent decades, although the underlying cause for this trend is not clear [2].

Clinical presentation

The shoulder girdle is often extremely swollen after proximal humeral fracture, with ecchymosis often tracking down the arm and into the chest. Because most patients who have proximal humeral fractures are elderly, assessment for concomitant injuries is paramount. Head injuries from the fall, cardiac or neurologic reasons for the fall, and other fractures are often first diagnosed at the initial evaluation for the shoulder injury.

Electromyographic evaluation has demonstrated that approximately two thirds (67%) of all patients who have proximal humeral fractures suffer acute neurologic injury from the violence of the injury. Most commonly, this involves either the axillary nerve (58%) or the suprascapular nerve (48%). Appreciation and documentation of this finding is important for prognostic evaluation and appropriate management of the injury.

Radiographic evaluation

Initial radiographic evaluation consists of the classic Neer trauma series with orthogonal views (anteroposterior, scapular "Y," or axillary views). Because of the anatomy of the proximal humerus, it may be difficult to appreciate fracture lines and fragment displacement. If plain radiographs do not offer adequate visualization, a CT scan with reconstructions may be necessary.

Classification

Neer's four-part classification system of proximal humerus fractures has endured by virtue of its simplicity. It allows for a conceptual understanding of the fracture pattern by dividing the fracture into separate parts. However, interobserver reliability and intraobserver reproducibility has been reported to be only poor to fair. Recently, a "comprehensive binary" description of fractures, based on Codman's original concept of fracture planes rather than fracture parts, has been described [3]. These fracture planes run along the old physeal lines of the proximal humerus. The system results in 12 possible fracture patterns: 6 patterns resulting in two fracture fragments, 5 patterns resulting in three fracture

* Corresponding author.
E-mail address: skrishnan@wbcarrellclinic.com (S.G. Krishnan).

doi:10.1016/j.hcl.2007.09.006

fragments, and 1 pattern resulting in four fracture fragments. This system has demonstrated improved interobserver reliability and better intraobserver reproducibility. The focus of this article is the evaluation and treatment of fractures of the proximal humerus in which four fracture fragments are involved.

Decision-making algorithm

Most proximal humerus fractures not involving four fracture segments are managed conservatively. However, after defining the fracture as one in which four fracture segments are involved, one must first assess the viability of the humeral head. Hertel [3] prospectively evaluated 100 intracapsular fractures of the proximal humerus for perfusion intraoperatively, by observation of backflow through a centrally placed borehole in the humeral head and by intraosseous laser Doppler. When combined with preoperative radiographs, ischemia of the humeral head correlated with posteromedial metaphyseal extension of less than 8 mm and disruption of the medial hinge, defined as displacement of the humeral shaft, of more than 2 mm. These two preoperative findings, in combination with an anatomic neck fracture, resulted in a 97% positive predictive value for humeral head ischemia. It is the authors' recommendation that four-part anatomic neck fractures with posteromedial metaphyseal extension of less than 8 mm and a medial hinge disruption of greater than 2 mm be treated with arthroplasty. On rare occasions, the medial hinge may be intact and indicate potential head viability, leading to management with osteosynthesis.

Surgical techniques

Osteosynthesis techniques

When the humeral head is deemed viable and fracture fixation is attempted, many methods of fracture fixation are available, each with inherent advantages and disadvantages. Percutaneous fixation can be performed with minimal soft tissue stripping and devascularization (Fig. 1). The largest reported peer-reviewed series on 27 three- and four-part proximal humerus fractures treated with percutaneous pin fixation demonstrated good to very good results in all three-part fractures at average 24-month follow-up [4]. The patients who had four-part fractures did not do as well, with 2 of the 18 patients eventually requiring revision to a prosthesis, 1 patient because of avascular necrosis and another for displacement.

When percutaneous techniques are not possible because of inadequate reduction or poor bone quality, proximal humeral plating allows for potentially greater control of, and ability to manipulate, individual fracture fragments into anatomic alignment (Fig. 2). This direct exposure comes at the cost of soft tissue stripping, which may lead to complications, and in osteoporotic bone, adequate fixation may be difficult. Recent advances in plate designs, such as proximal humeral locking plates, have renewed interest in this treatment option, and cadaveric studies demonstrate improved resistance to torsion in locking

A B

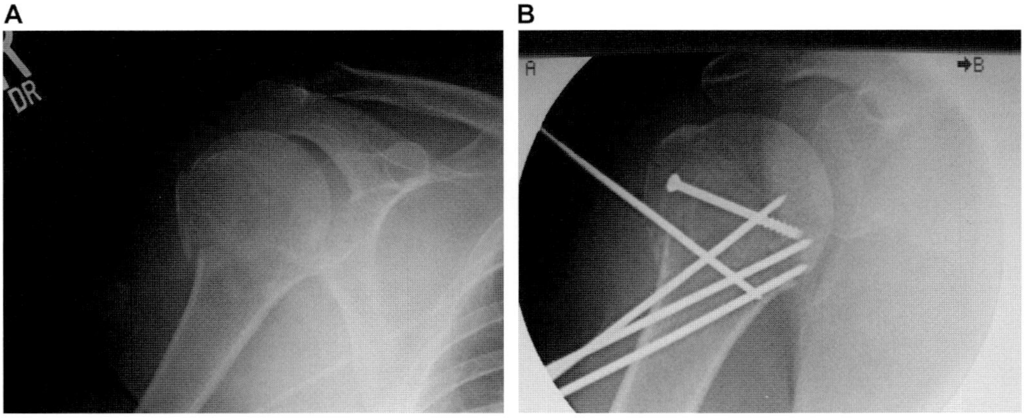

Fig. 1. (*A*) Preoperative anteroposterior radiograph of a proximal humerus fracture. (*B*) Postoperative anteroposterior radiograph of proximal humerus fracture treated with closed reduction and percutaneous pinning. (*From* Krishnan S, Sumant G, Pennington SD, et al. Shoulder arthroplasty for fracture: restoration of the "gothic arch". Techniques in Shoulder & Elbow Surgery 2005;6(2):57–66; with permission.)

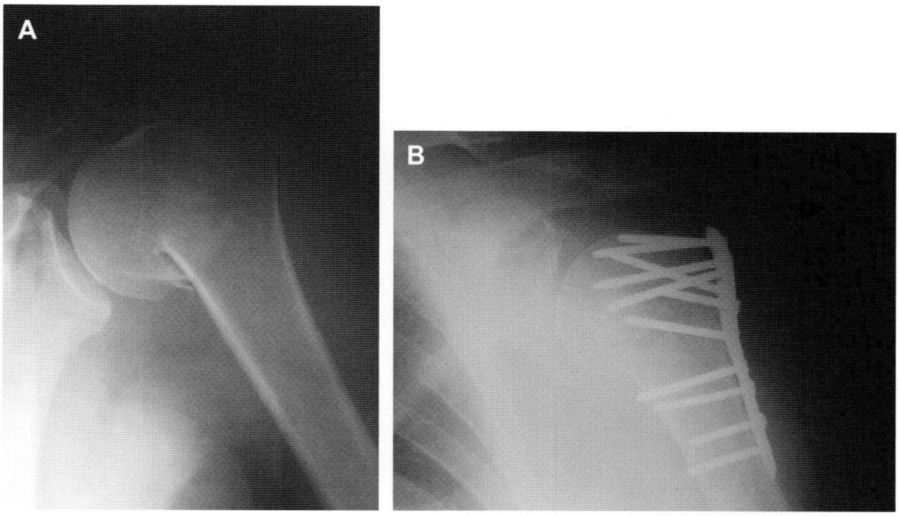

Fig. 2. (*A*) Preoperative anteroposterior radiograph of a proximal humerus fracture. (*B*) Postoperative anteroposterior radiograph of a proximal humerus fracture treated with locked-plating technique. (*From* Krishnan S, Sumant G, Pennington SD, et al. Shoulder arthroplasty for fracture: restoration of the "gothic arch". Techniques in Shoulder & Elbow Surgery 2005;6(2):57–66; with permission.)

plate constructs when compared with fixed angle blade plates [5]. These differences were particularly pronounced in osteoporotic specimens.

Intramedullary nails designed for proximal humeral fixation remain enticing but current designs still demonstrate higher postoperative dissatisfaction rates with rotator cuff pain and dysfunction. Hence, the authors do not advocate current intramedullary nailing techniques.

Shoulder arthroplasty for fracture

Primary hemiarthroplasty for fractures of the proximal humerus can result in good patient satisfaction and pain relief when osteosynthesis is not possible (Fig. 3). A recent retrospective review of 66 patients who underwent hemiarthroplasty for proximal humerus fracture demonstrated that 93% were pain free and satisfied with their results [6]. Other studies have also demonstrated successful pain relief but poorer functional outcomes with hemiarthroplasty, when compared with replacement arthroplasty performed for osteoarthritis.

Recent work has highlighted the importance of intraoperatively restoring anatomic humeral height, humeral version, and tuberosity reconstruction to improve outcomes after arthroplasty for shoulder fracture. The importance of anatomic repositioning of the tuberosities when performing hemiarthroplasty for proximal humeral fracture was demonstrated in a recent cadaveric study [7]. In these cadaveric shoulder specimens, four-part proximal humerus fractures were created and repaired with a shoulder hemiarthroplasty in which the tuberosities were intentionally positioned either anatomically or nonanatomically. The biomechanical effects of this tuberosity positioning demonstrated that anatomic repositioning of the tuberosities around a shoulder hemiarthroplasty produced external rotation kinematics identical to the native shoulder. When the tuberosities were malpositioned, however, an eightfold increase in torque was required to achieve the same degree of external rotation.

Clinical studies have also identified that failure to recreate proximal humeral anatomy when treating proximal humerus fractures with hemiarthroplasty can have negative clinical consequences [8]. In these studies, radiographic evidence of final tuberosity malpositioning correlated with poor functional results. Malpositioning of the prosthesis itself in turn correlated with tuberosity malposition. Boileau has pointed out the "unhappy triad" in which a prosthesis not only has excessive height but also is in excessive retroversion, and the greater tuberosity has been positioned too low. This combination was associated with poor functional results, persistent pain, and stiffness in all cases. It is clear from these studies that careful attention to the recreation of proximal humeral anatomy is critical in shoulder fracture arthroplasty.

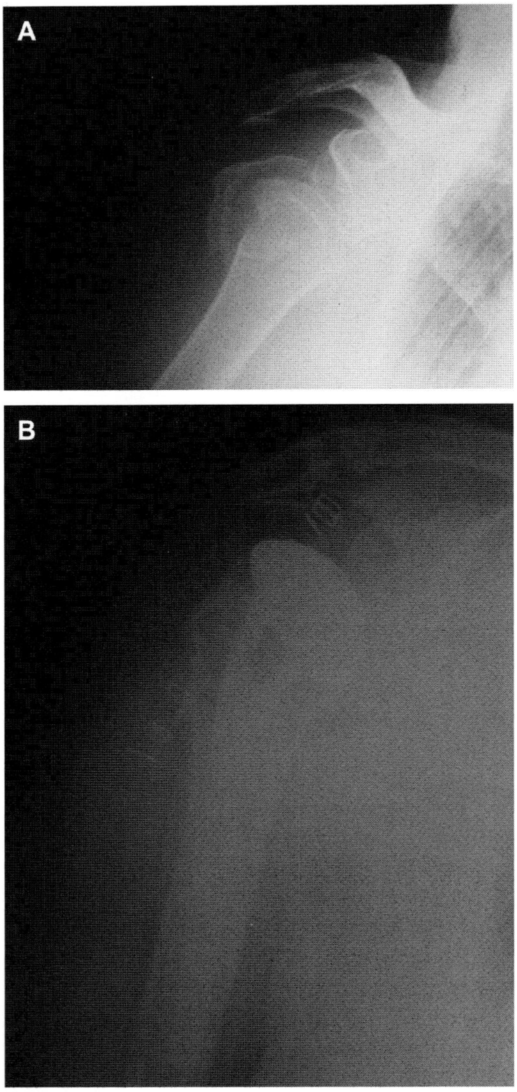

Fig. 3. (*A*) Preoperative anteroposterior radiograph of a proximal humerus fracture. (*B*) Postoperative anteroposterior radiograph of a proximal humerus fracture treated with proximal humeral hemiarthroplasty. (*From* Krishnan S, Sumant G, Pennington SD, et al. Shoulder arthroplasty for fracture: restoration of the "gothic arch". Techniques in Shoulder & Elbow Surgery 2005;6(2):57–66; with permission.)

The "Gothic arch" reconstruction

The "Gothic arch" is the authors' term for the architectural anatomy of the proximal shoulder girdle. The arch is easily seen on a normal radiograph by tracing the medial border of the proximal humeral calcar to the articular surface and joining this with the lateral border of the scapula to the articular surface; joining these lines forms the classical vaulted or Gothic arch shape seen in medieval period renaissance architecture (Fig. 4). Restoration of this Gothic arch provides a very reproducible technique for recreating proper humeral height and improving the potential for anatomic tuberosity reconstruction.

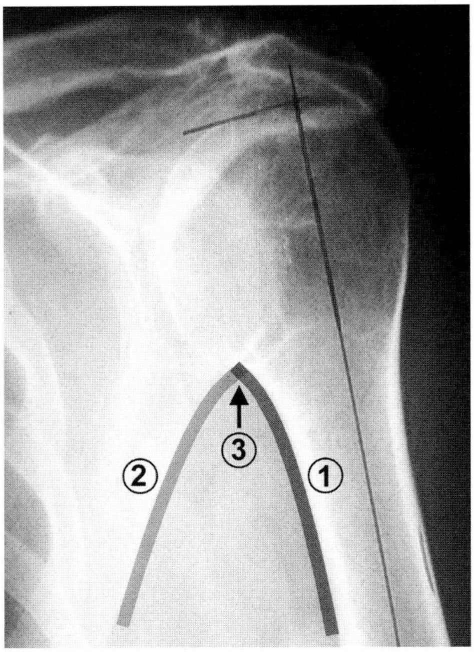

Fig. 4. Gothic arch of a normal shoulder girdle. (*1*) Outline of the medial border of the proximal humeral shaft (medial calcar) to the base of the humeral articular surface. (*2*) Outline of the lateral border of the scapula to the base of the glenoid articular surface. (*3*) Joining these lines creates a classical vaulted arch or Gothic arch shape. (*From* Krishnan S, Sumant G, Pennington SD, et al. Shoulder arthroplasty for fracture: restoration of the "gothic arch". Techniques in Shoulder & Elbow Surgery 2005;6(2):57–66; with permission.)

Preoperative radiographs are paramount in reproducible shoulder fracture arthroplasty and are used to determine the distance from the fracture line at the medial calcar to the desired height of the humeral head. By measuring the injury films and the contralateral humerus, an accurate assessment of humeral height can be made (Fig. 5). The authors obtain full-length scaled radiographs of the injured and the contralateral humeri with a ruler of defined length. These radiographs can even be done in the operating room immediately before surgery and should not be overlooked (Fig. 6). Although surgeons in the past have subjectively "eyeballed"

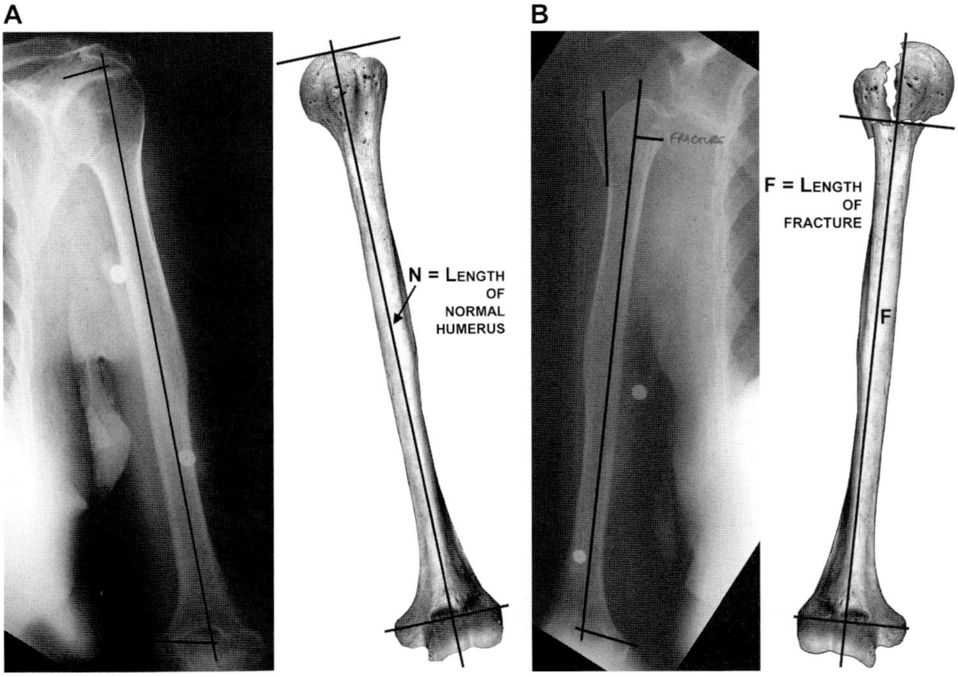

C

Calculations to Restore Gothic Arch

Normal side		**Fracture side**	
Ruler		**Ruler**	
Xray	11.2 cm	Xray	12.1 cm
Actual	10.0 cm	Actual	10.0 cm
Magnif.	1.12 cm	Magnif.	1.21 cm
Humeral length (N)		**Fx length (F)**	
Xray	35.0 cm	Xray	32.6 cm
Actual	31.3 cm	Actual	26.9 cm

Step 1. Fx to top of head: N - F = H
Actual N (31.3 cm) Minus Actual F (26.9 cm) Equals H (4.4 cm)

Step 2. Greater tuberosity length (G)
Xray 5.5 cm
Actual 4.5 cm (This number should be within 3-5 mm of fracture to top of head "H")

Fig. 5. (*A*) N = entire length of normal humerus along perpendicular from medial epicondyle to top of humeral head. Use scaled ruler on radiograph to calculate radiographic magnification and obtain actual number. (*B*) F = length of injured humerus along perpendicular from medial epicondyle to fracture at superior edge of medial calcar. Use scaled ruler on radiograph to calculate radiographic magnification and obtain actual number. (*From* Krishnan S, Sumant G, Pennington SD, et al. Shoulder arthroplasty for fracture: restoration of the "gothic arch". Techniques in Shoulder & Elbow Surgery 2005;6(2):57–66; with permission.) (*C*) N − F = H. H is the fracture to top of head height.

appropriate prosthetic position, this simple preparation allows an easy, reproducible, and accurate restoration of proximal humeral anatomy.

In addition, the authors also measure the length of the greater tuberosity fragment to ensure that humeral prosthetic height will allow for anatomic tuberosity reconstruction. This measurement is compared with the intraoperative length of the greater tuberosity fragment, which is perhaps the most important measurement because the greater tuberosity should sit 3 to 5 mm below the prosthetic head.

Restoration of the Gothic arch

The patient is placed in a modified beach-chair position, with the scapula supported. A 2.5- to

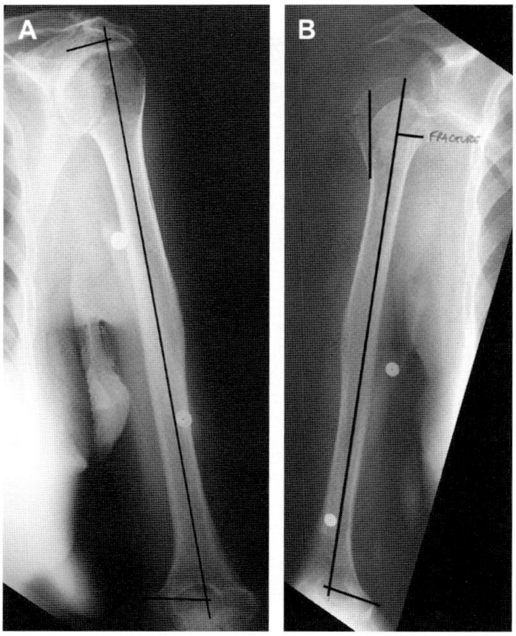

Fig. 6. (*A*) Scaled radiograph of normal humerus. (*B*) Scaled radiograph of injured humerus. (*From* Krishnan S, Sumant G, Pennington SD, et al. Shoulder arthroplasty for fracture: restoration of the "gothic arch". Techniques in Shoulder & Elbow Surgery 2005;6(2):57–66; with permission.)

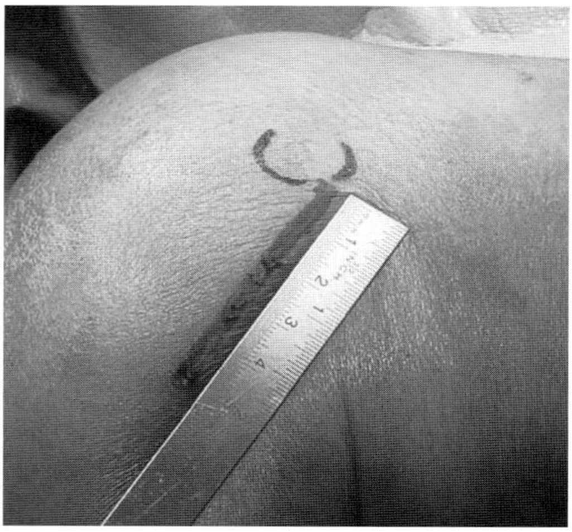

Fig. 7. Limited 3-in modified deltopectoral incision used for shoulder fracture arthroplasty. (*From* Krishnan S, Sumant G, Pennington SD, et al. Shoulder arthroplasty for fracture: restoration of the "gothic arch". Techniques in Shoulder & Elbow Surgery 2005;6(2):57–66; with permission.)

3-in deltopectoral approach is used. The authors have found that a well-placed incision and a mobile soft tissue window permits the procedure to be performed easily through this limited incision (Fig. 7). With adequate exposure, the fracture is visualized. Typically, the fracture line can be located with a blunt elevator or osteotome between the tuberosities, just posterior to the bicipital groove. Four horizontal mattress nonabsorbable sutures are placed around the greater tuberosity at the bone–tendon junction (two in the infraspinatus and two in the teres minor). Two temporary stay sutures are placed around the lesser tuberosity at the subscapularis/bone tendon junction. The tuberosities are gently retracted apart. The head fragment is removed and measured with a caliper. If the humeral head falls in between sizes, the smaller size is selected. Structural cancellous bone graft is procured from this articular fragment.

The medullary canal is prepared using cylindric reamers and fracture-specific trial implants (Aequalis Fracture Prosthesis, Tornier, St. Ismier, France) of increasing diameter by hand. Once the appropriate trial implant and head size are determined, retroversion is selected by facing the prosthetic head toward the glenoid with the forearm in neutral rotation at the side (approximately 20° of retroversion relative to the transepicondylar axis of the elbow).

The dedicated fracture-specific prosthetic stem of the appropriate diameter is opened and the preselected trial head is placed on this definitive implant with the eccentric head offset rotated into the most lateral position, which allows for the least amount of medial overhang of the humeral head during the all-important restoration of the Gothic arch.

This surgical technique differs from previously described techniques that reference the prosthetic humeral reconstruction off the lateral portion of the humerus and humeral metadiaphysis. In most proximal humeral fractures, the medial calcar of the proximal humerus is intact (this calcar is the proximal medial humeral shaft just inferior to the anatomic neck) (Fig. 8). In the few cases where the medial calcar is fractured, this fragment is often large and can be rigidly fixed with simple wire or heavy suture fixation. By referencing the reconstruction off the medial calcar, the Gothic arch can be recreated objectively in a methodic fashion (Fig. 9).

Using the preoperative radiographic calculations previously described, the appropriate mark

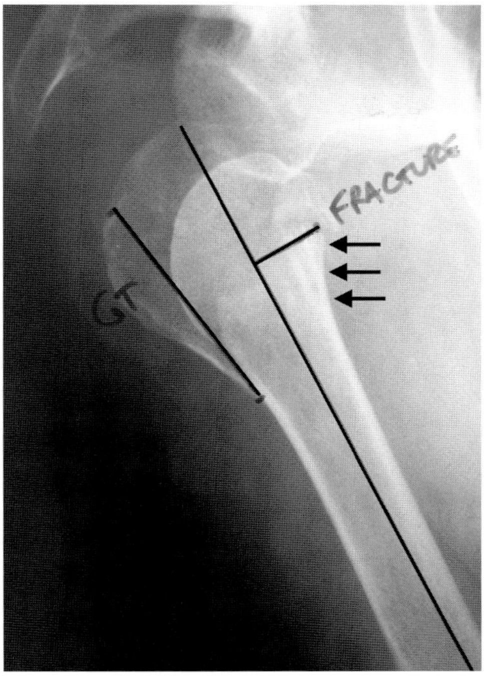

Fig. 8. Medial calcar (*arrows*) of the proximal humerus is the portion of the humeral shaft just below the inferior limit of the anatomic neck. (*From* Krishnan S, Sumant G, Pennington SD, et al. Shoulder arthroplasty for fracture: restoration of the "gothic arch". Techniques in Shoulder & Elbow Surgery 2005;6(2):57–66; with permission.)

is placed on the prosthetic implant and the implant is placed into the humeral shaft with the appropriately selected trial head. The lateral half of the Gothic arch (medial calcar of the humerus up to the inferior margin of the anatomic neck) should be unbroken (Fig. 10). If the arch is not "visualized," it will be for one of the following reasons:

- The prosthetic height is incorrect (usually too high).
- The medial calcar is fractured and has not been restored.
- The head size is either too large or has not been rotated into the most lateral offset position.

After establishing the arch, two drill holes are placed in the proximal humeral shaft before final prosthetic cementation. Two nonabsorbable sutures are placed in these holes in a horizontal mattress fashion to be used as tension-band sutures for final tuberosity osteosynthesis. The stem is cemented, using a standard third-generation technique, to the predetermined depth and rotation, in slight valgus. Three structural cancellous bone graft wedges that were previously obtained from the fractured humeral head are then placed as follows:

A

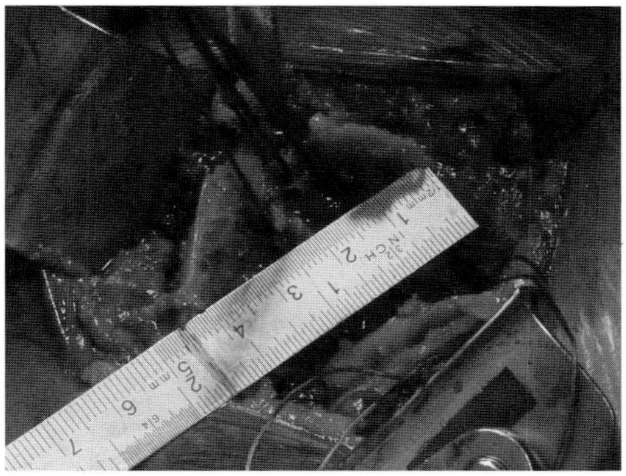

B

Calculations to Restore Gothic Arch

Normal side		**Fracture side**	
Ruler		**Ruler**	
Xray	11.2 cm	Xray	12.1 cm
Actual	10.0 cm	Actual	10.0 cm
Magnif.	1.12 cm	Magnif.	1.21 cm
Humeral length (N)		**Fx length (F)**	
Xray	35.0 cm	Xray	32.6 cm
Actual	31.3 cm	Actual	26.9 cm

Step 1. Fx to top of head: N - F = H
Actual N (31.3 cm) Minus Actual F (26.9 cm) Equals H (4.4 cm)

Step 2. Greater tuberosity length (G)
Xray 5.5 cm
Actual 4.5 cm (This number should be within 3-5 mm of fracture to top of head "H")

Step 3. Greater tuberosity measurement
Measurement 4.6 cm (This number should be within 5 mm of greater tuberosity length "G")

Fig. 9. (*A*) Greater tuberosity length (G) is measured and corrected for radiographic magnification using scale on radiograph. (*From* Krishnan S, Sumant G, Pennington SD, et al. Shoulder arthroplasty for fracture: restoration of the "gothic arch". Techniques in Shoulder & Elbow Surgery 2005;6(2):57–66; with permission.) (*B*) This number should be within 3 to 5 mm of the fracture to top of head height (H) that was marked on the prosthetic implant.

1. In the "window" of the fracture-specific prosthesis
2. Under the greater tuberosity at the lateral fin of the prosthesis
3. Under the medial edge of the prosthetic head between the head and neck of the implant

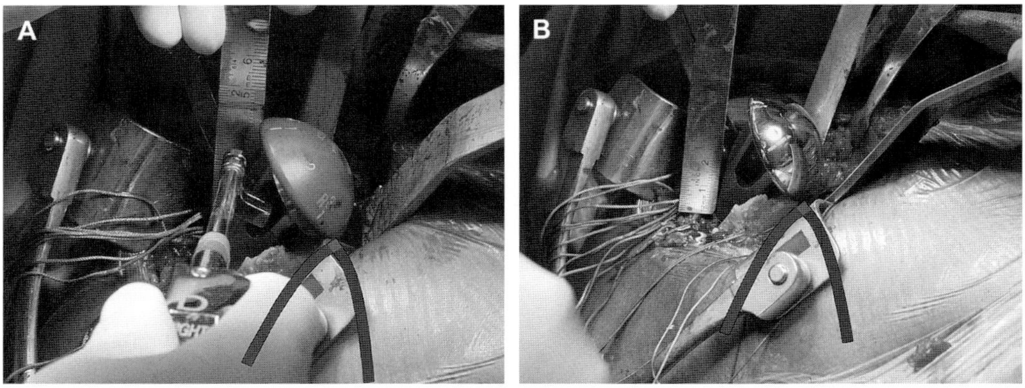

Fig. 10. (*A*) Gothic arch restoration with trial head on actual implant. Implant has been placed to predetermined mark and confirmed with ruler. (*B*) Final Gothic arch restoration. (*From* Krishnan S, Sumant G, Pennington SD, et al. Shoulder arthroplasty for fracture: restoration of the "gothic arch". Techniques in Shoulder & Elbow Surgery 2005;6(2): 57–66; with permission.)

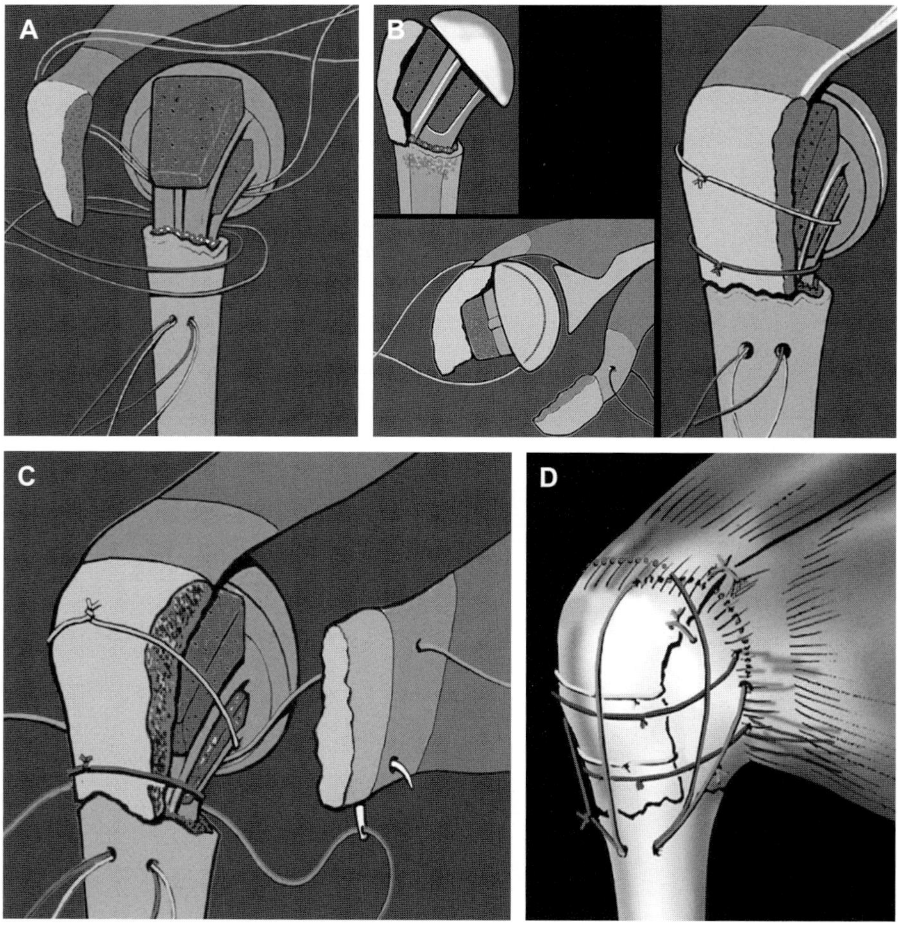

Fig. 11. (*A*) Six-suture configuration for anatomic tuberosity osteosynthesis. (*B*) Greater tuberosity fixation over lateral bone graft. (*C*) Lesser tuberosity fixation over medial bone graft. (*D*) Final tuberosity osteosynthesis with tension-band sutures passed through anterosuperior and posterosuperior cuff.

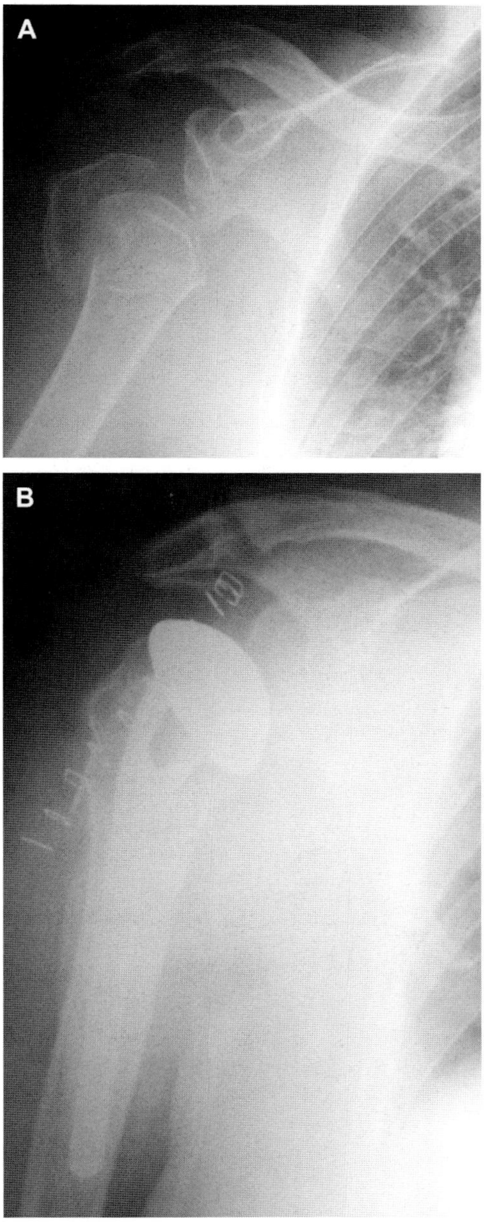

Fig. 12. (*A*) Four-part proximal humerus fracture with broken Gothic arch. (*B*) Restoration of the Gothic arch and anatomic tuberosity osteosynthesis. (*From* Krishnan S, Sumant G, Pennington SD, et al. Shoulder arthroplasty for fracture: restoration of the "gothic arch". Techniques in Shoulder & Elbow Surgery 2005;6(2):57–66; with permission.)

Tuberosity osteosynthesis is performed as described elsewhere, and the biceps is tenodesed within the intertubercular groove/rotator interval to soft tissue (Fig. 11) [8,9]. The shoulder is placed through a full range of motion, to ensure no micromotion of the tuberosity fragments. Passive intraoperative range of motion should be at least 160° of elevation, 40° of external rotation, and 70° of internal rotation. Postoperative radiographs should demonstrate anatomic reconstruction of the proximal humerus (Fig. 12).

Postoperatively, patients are placed into a SmartSling orthosis (Innovation Sports, Ossur, California) for 6 weeks. Immediate supine passive motion is begun the day after surgery, with motion limits dictated by the intraoperative evaluation following tuberosity osteosynthesis. Active motion is allowed at 7 weeks after surgery. Resistance exercises begin 10 weeks after surgery.

Clinical results after shoulder arthroplasty for fracture

Using this approach, the authors have retrospectively reviewed 130 consecutive patients who had proximal humerus fractures who underwent the Gothic arch technique for fracture arthroplasty at minimum 2-year follow-up. Mean active anterior elevation was 129° (range 50–165), mean American Shoulder and Elbow Society (ASES) score was 74 (range 10–100), and 114 (88%) greater tuberosities healed anatomically. Pain scores averaged 1.2 (0 = no pain; 10 = worst pain). Satisfaction averaged 9.1 (0 = unsatisfied; 10 = completely satisfied). For patients with active anterior elevation (AAE) greater than 120° (106 cases), mean age was 62 years, mean AAE was 146°, mean ASES score was 86, and 94% of tuberosities healed. Those with AAE less than 120° (24 cases) had mean age of 82 years, mean AAE of 95°, mean ASES score of 46, and 61% of tuberosities healed ($P < .03$). For patients who had fracture-specific prosthesis (65 cases), mean AAE was 140°, mean ASES score was 82, and 92% of tuberosities healed ($P < .05$) [10,11].

Summary

Four-part proximal humerus fractures represent a difficult entity in the management of upper extremity trauma. Most of these fractures are not amenable to operative fixation; thus, surgical address is necessarily one of fracture arthroplasty. Timely reestablishment of the Gothic arch using a fracture-specific prosthesis leads reliably to anatomic tuberosity osteosynthesis. Hence, shoulder arthroplasty for fracture should be considered an augmented osteosynthesis, with precise prosthetic implantation supplementing anatomic tuberosity reconstruction. Further investigations are ongoing regarding the use of specific fracture implants and biologic substrates in an attempt to improve further the rate of tuberosity healing in the older patient population after this operation.

References

[1] Nordqvist A, Petersson CJ. Incidence and causes of shoulder girdle injuries in an urban population. J Shoulder Elbow Surg 1995;4(2):107–12.

[2] Palvanen M, Kannus P, Niemi S, et al. Update in the epidemiology of proximal humeral fractures. Clin Orthop Relat Res 2006;442:87–92.

[3] Hertel R, Hempfing A, Stiehler M, et al. Predictors of humeral head ischemia after intracapsular fracture of the proximal humerus. J Shoulder Elbow Surg 2004;13(4):427–33, 3.

[4] Resch H, Povacz P, Frohlich R, et al. Percutaneous fixation of three- and four-part fractures of the proximal humerus. J Bone Joint Surg Br 1997;79(2): 295–300.

[5] Weinstein DM, Bratton DR, Ciccone WJ 2nd, et al. Locking plates improve torsional resistance in the stabilization of three-part proximal humeral fractures. J Shoulder Elbow Surg 2006;15(2):239–43.

[6] Mighell MA, Kolm GP, Collinge CA, et al. Outcomes of hemiarthroplasty for fractures of the proximal humerus. J Shoulder Elbow Surg 2003;12(6):569–77.

[7] Frankle MA, Greenwald DP, Markee BA, et al. Biomechanical effects of malposition of tuberosity fragments on the humeral prosthetic reconstruction for four-part proximal humerus fractures. J Shoulder Elbow Surg 2001;10(4):321–6.

[8] Boileau P, Krishnan SG, Tinsi L, et al. Tuberosity malposition and migration: reasons for poor outcomes after hemiarthroplasty for displaced fractures of the proximal humerus. J Shoulder Elbow Surg 2002;11(5):401–12.

[9] Boileau P, Walch G, Krishnan SG. Tuberosity osteosynthesis and hemiarthroplasty for four-part fractures of the proximal humerus. Techniques in Shoulder and Elbow Surgery 2000;1:96–109.

[10] Krishnan SG, Lin KC, Burkhead WZ. Shoulder arthroplasty for fracture: results of the Gothic arch technique and a fracture-specific prosthesis. American Shoulder and Elbow Surgeons, Specialty Day Proceedings, San Diego (CA), 2007.

[11] Krishnan S, Sumant G, Pennington SD, et al. Shoulder arthroplasty for fracture: restoration of the "gothic arch". Techniques in Shoulder & Elbow Surgery 2005;6(2):57–66.

ELSEVIER
SAUNDERS

Hand Clin 23 (2007) 425–430

HAND
CLINICS

Reverse Shoulder Arthroplasty for the Treatment of Proximal Humeral Fractures

Bryan Wall, MD[a,*], Gilles Walch, MD[b]

[a]The CORE Institute, 14420 West Meeker Boulevard, Suite 300, Sun City West, AZ 85375, USA
[b]Centre Orthopédique Santy, 24 Avenue Paul Santy, Lyon, France 69008

Proximal humeral fractures account for up to 5% of all fractures seen in emergency departments in some series [1]. These fracture patterns are difficult for the surgeon to manage and often result in significant long-term disability for the patient. Complex fractures occur frequently in elderly patients who often have comorbidities [1]. As our population ages, these complex fractures are expected to be seen much more frequently. The incidence of these fractures may triple in the decades to come [2].

Proximal humeral fractures are classified most commonly according to the system devised by Neer [3]. In recent years, the treatment of displaced three- and four-part fractures of the proximal humerus has elicited significant interest. The loss of function of an extremity can impair the ability to perform the simplest activities of daily living and threaten one's ability to live independently.

Evaluation

The examination of the patient who has a complex proximal humeral fracture should include a detailed neurovascular status of the extremity. Axillary and suprascapular nerve palsies are frequently seen if electromyography is performed. Nearly all of these will recover spontaneously, but the presence of a palsy may delay recovery and rehabilitation [4].

Plain radiographs of the affected shoulder often allow classification of the fracture pattern according to Neer [5]. Concern about the reliability of plain films alone has led some to recommend routine CT scans to depict the anatomy and classify the fracture pattern more accurately [6].

Treatment options

Several variables must be taken into account when devising a treatment plan for the patient who has a complex proximal humerus fracture. Patient age, general health, bone quality, and functional expectations should all be considered when setting goals for fracture treatment. An elderly patient who lives alone with few other medical conditions may be treated more aggressively than a younger patient with severe comorbid disease who already requires significant assistance.

Nonoperative treatment

Nonoperative treatment has been traditionally reserved for patients who were either too ill to undergo surgery or who had extremely limited functional demands. Although a few investigators have reported good patient satisfaction without surgery, the functional results of nonoperative treatment are almost universally poor [7–10]. In a review of the literature, Compito and colleagues [11] showed that only 5% of patients undergoing nonoperative treatment could expect satisfactory results. In a separate literature review, Misra and colleagues [12] showed greater pain and inferior function in patients managed nonoperatively, when compared with those treated with internal fixation or hemiarthroplasty.

* Corresponding author.
E-mail address: bryan.wall@thecoreinstitute.com (B. Wall).

doi:10.1016/j.hcl.2007.08.002

hand.theclinics.com

When nonoperative treatment is undertaken, the arm is most commonly placed in a sling for a period of approximately 2 weeks. After this initial period, pendulum exercise can be begun. Therapy then progresses according to fracture healing, as determined by clinical examination and radiographic signs of callus formation.

The risk of severe complication with conservative management is minimal. Nonunion or malunion of the tuberosities occurs in almost all cases [7]. Careful consideration must be given to the long-term consequences of nonoperative treatment. Patients who have pre-existing malunion or nonunion who undergo revision to a hemiarthroplasty tend to have poor functional outcomes when compared with patients who are managed with immediate surgery [13,14].

Internal fixation

Reduction of the fracture fragments, in addition to some form of internal fixation, is an attractive concept. When done through a deltopectoral approach, fixation techniques include the use of plates, intramedullary rods sometimes augmented by tension bands. Less aggressive fixation options include isolated tension bands using wire or sutures, interfragmentary screws, or Kirschner wires. Unfortunately, the additional surgical trauma may disrupt any remaining blood supply to the articular fragment and these patients often go on to osteonecrosis [9,15]. Although late osteonecrosis does not ensure a poor result, revision to hemiarthroplasty after failed fixation gives poor results, when compared with patients undergoing hemiarthroplasty at the time of fracture [15,16]. Good results using internal fixation methods are often reported in younger patients who have better bone quality and in valgus-impacted fractures that allow minimal surgical hardware [17–19].

Hemiarthroplasty

Many investigators have recommended hemiarthroplasty in the acute setting after a fracture [9,10]. Pain relief is normally good, and hemiarthroplasty eliminates the chance of late osteonecrosis. Despite these advantages, functional outcomes are often disappointing [20–22].

Poor functional results can be related to a number of factors. The relative rarity of these fractures and surgeon inexperience may play a role. Many of these older patients are in poor health. Women over the age of 75 have been shown to fare worse than average [20]. Radiographic evidence of tuberosity malunion or nonunion may predict poor outcomes. Accurate reconstruction of the normal height and retroversion of the proximal humerus is exceedingly difficult, even in experienced hands. Boileau and Bigliani [20] have separately identified problems with tuberosity osteosynthesis as the most important factors associated with poor results. Tanner and Cofield [23] noted that tuberosity displacement was the most common postoperative complication of proximal humeral arthroplasty after an acute fracture. This problem is magnified in the elderly patient who has severely osteoporotic bone. In many cases, the quality of the tuberosities is poor, and resorption can occur, despite anatomic positioning, bone grafting, and satisfactory osteosynthesis.

In response to this problem, fracture-specific stems have been designed to help maximize tuberosity healing potential by removing unnecessary metal from the proximal portion of the implant and allowing for better bone grafting and bony apposition. Fracture jigs that quantify humeral height and retroversion have been designed in an attempt to replicate normal humeral anatomy better [24,25]. Although these newer devices show some promise, objective reports of their effectiveness are still lacking.

Reverse shoulder arthroplasty

Reverse shoulder arthroplasty offers some potential benefits over traditional hemiarthroplasty in the setting of acute three- and four-part fractures. The implant is designed to allow for active arm elevation in the face of a dysfunctional cuff. Healing of the greater tuberosity may improve active motion, especially external rotation. However, if tuberosity malunion occurs, the patient should retain at least some active elevation. The less intensive rehabilitation protocols for reverse arthroplasty also allow for earlier motion than can be obtained with hemiarthroplasty.

Patient selection

Proper patient selection for reverse shoulder arthroplasty is important. Patient age should be a consideration. In most series reported for the reverse prosthesis, the mean age of the patient group is nearly 70 or older [26–28]. Little data are currently available on long-term function and loosening rates, and currently, no detailed series are focusing on younger patients [29]. With these factors in mind, it would seem prudent to restrict the routine use of reverse shoulder arthroplasty for acute fracture treatment to older patients.

Patient factors which can be predictors of tuberosity migration should be examined. Those who are in poor health, are osteoporotic, and may have difficulty healing should be approached with caution when contemplating internal fixation or hemiarthroplasty. Women over the age of 75 are at particular risk for tuberosity complications [20] because of the osteoporotic nature of the proximal humeral bone, and other factors that negatively impact bone quality may have a similar effect.

The status of the patient's rotator cuff should also be taken into account. Pre-existing and concomitant tears may be difficult to address in the elderly patient, secondary to the quality of the cuff and bony tissues.

Surgical technique

Reverse shoulder arthroplasty can be performed through either a standard deltopectoral approach or a superolateral approach. The deltopectoral approach offers several advantages, including no division of the deltoid muscle, which may allow for easier postoperative rehabilitation; the approach allows exposure of the entire humerus in the unusual case of a fracture that extends into the humeral shaft; the glenoid sphere can be placed more inferiorly on the glenoid face, perhaps decreasing the rate of scapular notching [30]. The main advantage of the superolateral approach has been a decreased rate of instability [31], which is thought to be because the anterior-inferior capsule and the subscapularis are not dissected using this approach. After a fracture in which the lesser tuberosity is displaced from the humeral shaft and greater tuberosity, this advantage would seem to be less important.

The glenoid sphere is placed just inferior to the center of the glenoid, so that the inferior edge of the sphere is approximately 3 to 4 mm inferior to the inferior edge of the glenoid, which is thought to decrease the amount of mechanical impingement between the humeral component and the inferior border of the glenoid, thereby decreasing scapular notching (Fig. 1).

The appropriate humeral length for restoration may be difficult to judge. The tuberosities can be used to attempt to replicate the level of the original joint surface. The inferior-medial portion of the neck, if intact, can also be a useful reference. The most important consideration should be the amount of tension across the joint. The glenoid sphere and the humeral cup should have essentially no pistoning between them, and the tension of the deltoid should be adequate to hold the joint reduced. If this is not the case after

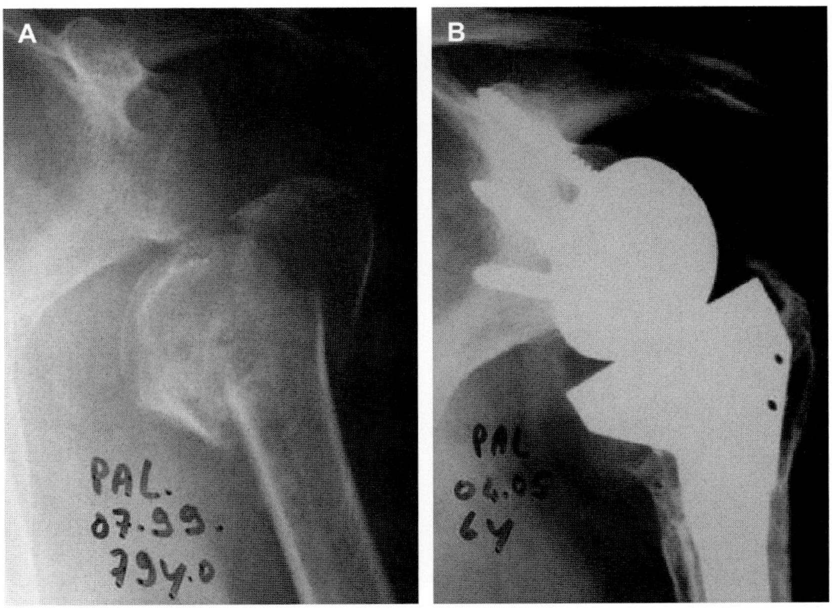

Fig. 1. (*A*) Four-part fracture with significant greater tuberosity displacement. (*B*) Tuberosity healing occurred after suture fixation around the prosthesis.

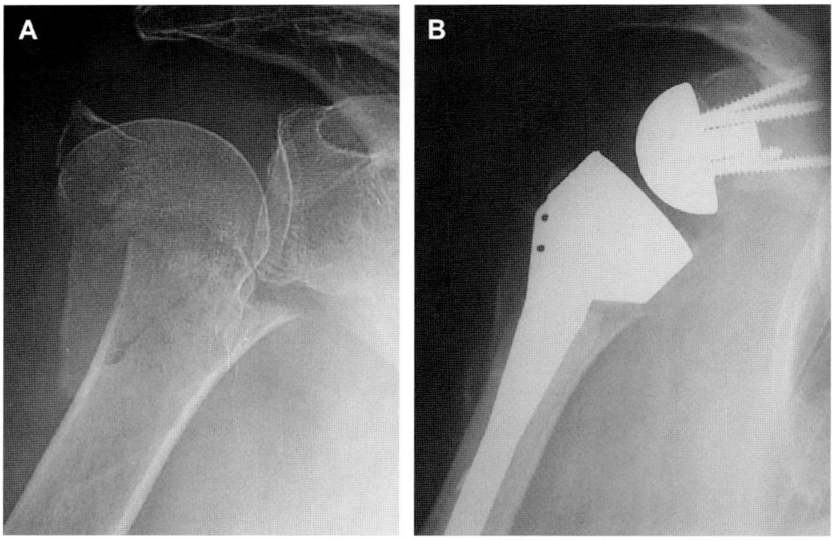

Fig. 2. (*A*) Four-part fracture in an 81-year-old female patient who had extension into the proximal humeral diaphysis treated using a reverse prosthesis. (*B*) A metallic spacer was used to increase the tension of the deltoid.

the humeral component is implanted, either a thicker polyethylene insert or a modular metallic spacer should be used to increase tension to appropriate levels (Fig. 2).

The authors' preference is to use a cemented humeral stem, although press-fit designs are available. With some modular implants, it is possible to use a cemented humeral stem with a press-fit metaphyseal segment, which may allow for better tuberosity fixation to the proximal portion of the implant, but the concept is unproven.

The correct amount of retroversion to use when implanting the humeral component is controversial. When implanting a reverse prosthesis for cuff tear arthropathy, recommendations have ranged from no retroversion to up to 30° of retroversion, and have not been based on any significant data. To date, no study convincingly proves that any particular degree of retroversion is better for joint stability or motion. It is the authors' preference to place the component in the degree of retroversion that provides the maximal amount of surrounding bone to the metaphysis of the implant, which normally places the implant between 0° and 20° of retroversion. This placement may be more difficult to appreciate in the fracture setting.

Once the prosthesis is in place, the tuberosities can be sutured to one another around it, which is done using a heavy, nonabsorbable suture. Vertical sutures can be added to help augment the stability of the repair. Currently, no comparative studies examine the potential benefits of tuberosity fixation after fracture. Compelling evidence shows that function and external rotation are improved in cuff tear arthropathy patients who have an intact teres minor [32]. In addition, internal rotation is improved in this patient group when subscapularis is sufficient to repair after prosthesis implantation [26].

Postoperative rehabilitation

Postoperative immobilization normally consists of immobilization in a sling for 3 weeks, with only pendulum exercises. Patients then begin progressive motion as tolerated. The postoperative rehabilitation and immobilization are typically less intensive than for patients undergoing hemiarthroplasty. Elderly patients may have a difficult time with a more demanding protocol. In a study by Boileau and colleagues [20], 30% of patients older than 80 were unable to tolerate the postoperative protocol for fracture hemiarthroplasty. This protocol can be modified as needed, based on the quality of tuberosity fixation and the patient's ability to tolerate the postoperative regimen.

Results

To date, reports of the reverse prosthesis being used for acute fractures have been limited, and most are small series [26,33]. Bufquin and colleagues [34] reported on a consecutive series of 43 patients with a mean follow-up of 22 months. Mean active elevation was found to be 97° and the Constant score averaged 44 points. Displacement of one or both of the tuberosities occurred in 53% of patients. Tuberosity healing had no effect on clinical results. They noted complications in 12 cases, with transient neurologic complications being the most common. One patient experienced a dislocation.

Cazeneuve and Cristofari have published a report of 16 proximal humeral fractures with similar conclusions. They were able to obtain tuberosity healing in just five cases, yet the mean final Constant score was 60, compared with a score of 83 for the unaffected shoulder. The study cited four complications, with only one dislocation [35].

Summary

The reverse prosthesis was originally designed for patients with cuff-tear arthropathy and has performed well in larger studies of that patient population [26–28]. With this initial success, indications for reverse shoulder arthroplasty have expanded to include other conditions with deficient cuff tissue or abnormal rotator cuff function. It has been used successfully in post-traumatic arthritis, proximal humeral malunion, revision of failed shoulder arthroplasty, and tumor reconstruction [26,36–38].

The role for reverse shoulder arthroplasty in the treatment of acute proximal humeral fractures is not fully established. Although early studies are encouraging, they have not shown superior results to more traditional treatments. The ability of the reverse prosthesis to compensate for tuberosity malunion makes it an attractive choice. It would seem prudent to consider reverse shoulder arthroplasty in those patients most likely to have problems with tuberosity healing, including the elderly and women. In the authors' current practices, they strongly consider reverse shoulder arthroplasty in all patients older than 75. Younger patients are included if they have specific factors that may impair tuberosity healing.

The next step in the evolution of proximal humeral fracture treatment will require prospective, randomized studies to determine which patient groups derive any benefit from reverse shoulder arthroplasty. Additional studies are required to determine the necessity for tuberosity fixation, proper humeral version, proper humeral height, and appropriate postoperative rehabilitation. Until this information is available, reverse shoulder arthroplasty should be used judiciously in the treatment of complex proximal humeral fractures.

References

[1] Horak J, Nilsson BE. Epidemiology of fracture of the upper end of the humerus. Clin Orthop Relat Res 1975;112:250–3.
[2] Palvanen M, Kannus P, Niemi S, et al. Update in the epidemiology of proximal humeral fractures. Clin Orthop Relat Res 2006;442:87–92.
[3] Neer CS. Displaced proximal humeral fractures. I. Classification and evaluation. J Bone Joint Surg 1970;52(6):1077–89.
[4] Visser CP, Coene LN, Brand R, et al. Nerve lesions in proximal humeral fractures. J Shoulder Elbow Surg 2001;10(5):421–7.
[5] Shrader MW, Sanchez-Sotelo J, Sperling JW, et al. Understanding proximal humerus fractures: image analysis, classification, and treatment. J Shoulder Elbow Surg 2005;14(5):497–505.
[6] Brien H, Noftall F, MacMaster S, et al. Neer's classification system: a critical appraisal. J Trauma 1995; 38(2):257–60.
[7] Zyto K, Ahrengart L, Sperber A, et al. Treatment of displaced proximal humeral fractures in elderly patients. J Bone Joint Surg Br 1997;79(3):412–7.
[8] Zyto K. Non-operative treatment of comminuted fractures of the proximal humerus in elderly patients. Injury 1998;29(5):349–52.
[9] Neer CS. Displaced proximal humeral fractures. II. Treatment of three-part and four-part displacement. J Bone Joint Surg Am 1970;52(6):1090–103.
[10] Stableforth PG. Four-part fractures of the neck of the humerus. J Bone Joint Surg Br 1984;66(1):104–8.
[11] Compito CA, Self EB, Bigliani LU. Arthroplasty and acute shoulder trauma. Reasons for success and failure. Clin Orthop Relat Res 1994;307:27–36.
[12] Misra A, Kapur R, Maffulli N. Complex proximal humeral fractures in adults–a systematic review of management. Injury 2001;32(5):363–72.
[13] Beredjiklian PK, Iannotti JP, Norris TR, et al. Operative treatment of malunion of a fracture of the proximal aspect of the humerus. J Bone Joint Surg Am 1998;80(10):1484–97.
[14] Norris TR, Green A, McGuigan FX. Late prosthetic shoulder arthroplasty for displaced proximal humerus fractures. J Shoulder Elbow Surg 1995; 4(4):271–80.
[15] Schai P, Imhoff A, Preiss S. Comminuted humeral head fractures: a multicenter analysis. J Shoulder Elbow Surg 1995;4(5):319–30.
[16] Gerber C, Hersche O, Berberat C. The clinical relevance of posttraumatic avascular necrosis of the humeral head. J Shoulder Elbow Surg 1998;7(6): 586–90.

[17] Resch H, Beck E, Bayley I. Reconstruction of the valgus-impacted humeral head fracture. J Shoulder Elbow Surg 1995;4(2):73–80.
[18] Jaberg H, Warner JJ, Jakob RP. Percutaneous stabilization of unstable fractures of the humerus. J Bone Joint Surg Am 1992;74(4):508–15.
[19] Jakob RP, Miniaci A, Anson PS, et al. Four-part valgus impacted fractures of the proximal humerus. J Bone Joint Surg Br 1991;73(2):295–8.
[20] Boileau P, Krishnan SG, Tinsi L, et al. Tuberosity malposition and migration: reasons for poor outcomes after hemiarthroplasty for displaced fractures of the proximal humerus. J Shoulder Elbow Surg 2002;11(5):401–12.
[21] Goldman RT, Koval KJ, Cuomo F, et al. Functional outcome after humeral head replacement for acute three- and four-part proximal humeral fractures. J Shoulder Elbow Surg 1995;4(2):81–6.
[22] Prakash U, McGurty DW, Dent JA. Hemiarthroplasty for severe fractures of the proximal humerus. J Shoulder Elbow Surg 2002;11(5):428–30.
[23] Tanner MW, Cofield RH. Prosthetic arthroplasty for fractures and fracture-dislocations of the proximal humerus. Clin Orthop Relat Res 1983;179:116–28.
[24] Boileau P, Walch G. Hemiprosthetic replacement in fractures of the proximal humerus. Semin Arthroplasty 2000;11:54–70.
[25] Boileau P, Walch G. Shoulder arthroplasty for fractures: problems and solutions. In: Walch G, Boileau P, editors. Shoulder arthroplasty. Heidelberg (Germany): Springer-Verlag; 1999. p. 297–314.
[26] Wall B, Nové-Josserand L, O'Connor DP, et al. Reverse total shoulder arthroplasty: a review of results according to etiology. J Bone Joint Surg Am 2007; 89(7):1476–85.
[27] Frankle M, Siegal S, Pupello D, et al. The reverse shoulder prosthesis for glenohumeral arthritis associated with severe rotator cuff deficiency. A minimum two-year follow-up study of sixty patients. J Bone Joint Surg Am 2005;87(8):1697–705.
[28] Werner CM, Steinmann PA, Gilbart M, et al. Treatment of painful pseudoparesis due to irreparable rotator cuff dysfunction with the Delta III reverse-ball-and-socket total shoulder prosthesis. J Bone Joint Surg Am 2005;87(7):1476–86.
[29] Guery J, Favard L, Sirveaux F, et al. Reverse total shoulder arthroplasty. Survivorship analysis of eighty replacements followed for five to ten years. J Bone Joint Surg Am 2006;88(8):1742–7.
[30] Simovitch RW, Zumstein MA, Lohri E, et al. Predictors of scapular notching in patients managed with the Delta III reverse total shoulder replacement. J Bone Joint Surg Am 2007;89(3):588–600.
[31] Wall B, Nové-Josserand L, Walch G. Instability of the reverse prosthesis [abstract 312]. In: Proceedings of the American Academy of Orthopaedic Surgeons. San Diego; 2007. p. 582–3.
[32] Simovitch RW, Helmy N, Zumstein MA, et al. Impact of fatty infiltration of the teres minor muscle on the outcome of reverse total shoulder arthroplasty. J Bone Joint Surg Am 2007;89(5):934–9.
[33] Sirveaux F, Navez G, Favard L, et al. Reverse prosthesis for acute proximal humerus fracture, the multicentric study. In: Walch G, Boileau P, Molé D, et al, editors. Reverse shoulder arthroplasty: clinical results, complications, revision. Montpellier, France: Sauramps Médical; 2006. p. 73–80.
[34] Bufquin T, Hersan A, Hubert L, et al. Reverse shoulder arthroplasty for the treatment of three- and four-part fractures of the proximal humerus in the elderly: a prospective review of 43 cases with a short-term follow-up. J Bone Joint Surg Br 2007;89(4):516–20.
[35] Cazeneuve JF, Cristofari DJ. Grammont reversed prosthesis for acute complex fracture of the proximal humerus in an elderly population with 5 to 12 years follow-up. Rev Chir Orthop Reparatrice Appar Mot 2006;92(6):543–8 [in French].
[36] Boileau P, Watkinson D, Hatzidakis AM, et al. Neer Award 2005: The Grammont reverse shoulder prosthesis: results in cuff tear arthritis, fracture sequelae, and revision arthroplasty. J Shoulder Elbow Surg 2006;15(5):527–40.
[37] Levy J, Frankle M, Mighell M, et al. The use of the reverse shoulder prosthesis for the treatment of failed hemiarthroplasty for proximal humeral fracture. J Bone Joint Surg Am 2007;89(2):292–300.
[38] De Wilde L, Sys G, Julien Y, et al. The reversed Delta shoulder prosthesis in reconstruction of the proximal humerus after tumour resection. Acta Orthop Belg 2003;69(6):495–500.

ELSEVIER
SAUNDERS

Hand Clin 23 (2007) 431–435

HAND
CLINICS

Proximal Humerus and Humeral Shaft Fractures in Children

M. Wade Shrader, MD

The CORE Institute, 19841 N. 27th Avenue, Suite 108, Phoenix, AZ 85027, USA

Proximal humerus fractures

Proximal humerus fractures in children are relatively rare in terms of the overall prevalence of pediatric fractures. The incidence is about 1 to 3 cases/1000 population per year, compromising fewer than 5% of all pediatric fractures [1,2]. Proximal humerus fractures occur either in the metaphysis or through the physis. Physeal fractures of the proximal humerus represent fewer than 3% of all physeal fractures [1] and may occur in children of any age, but occur more commonly in adolescents. Fractures of the proximal humeral metaphysis occur more often in small children, whereas adolescents usually fracture through the physis. A proximal humerus fracture is also a common birth-related injury in neonates [3].

One of the most important features of these fractures is their ability to remodel. This remodeling capability is primarily due to the thick periosteum in this anatomic location and the relatively close proximity of the physis [4]. Thus, significant displacements and angulations are often acceptable for these injuries, with even moderately displaced and angulated fractures healing without significant residual cosmetic or functional deficits.

History and physical examination

The mechanism of injury usually occurs as a result of a fall on an outstretched hand, or a direct blow to the lateral aspect of the shoulder. These fractures are frequently adolescent sports injuries. It has been estimated that approximately 50% of all shoulder girdle fractures (including clavicle fractures) occur during sporting activities [5]. High-contact sports that have a relatively high risk include football, hockey, gymnastics, and horseback riding.

Proximal humerus fractures can occur in neonates as a result of birth trauma. These fractures are often caused by rotation or hyperextension of the extremity during passage through the birth canal, and are often associated with shoulder dystocia or breech presentation. However, presentation and prenatal size have not been found to be statistically significant predictors for perinatal fracture [6].

Proximal humerus fractures in otherwise healthy infants can be a red flag for nonaccidental trauma or child abuse. Because no specific fracture pattern is pathonomic for abuse in proximal humerus fractures, clinical suspicion should remain high when evaluating children with these injuries. Although the exact mechanism in nonaccidental trauma is often unknown, one frequent fracture mechanism is a twisting injury.

Fractures that occur in older children with a minimal history of trauma are a red flag to be aware of a pathologic fracture, because unicameral bone cysts are common in this area [7]. The differential diagnosis of a nonverbal young child includes proximal humerus fracture, osteomyelitis or septic arthritis, and brachial plexus palsy.

The child typically presents with severe shoulder pain and a history of a fall or traumatic event. For nondisplaced fractures, the physical findings may be limited to tenderness and mild swelling [8]. For displaced fractures, the arm is often shortened and held in extension. The displaced distal fragment may cause a prominence anteriorly. The proximal fragment is usually well centered in the glenoid fossa, but it is abducted and externally

E-mail address: wshrader@thecoreinstitute.com

0749-0712/07/$ - see front matter
doi:10.1016/j.hcl.2007.09.002

rotated because of the forces from the rotator cuff. The distal fragment is displaced anteriorly from the unopposed action of the pectoralis major and latissimus dorsi.

Imaging

In general, any child with complaints of shoulder pain should have plain radiographs. However, the proximal humeral physis does not appear radiographically until about 6 months of age, so these films may be nondiagnostic in the neonatal period. Ultrasound may be helpful in the assessment of infants. Usually, plain radiographs are all that is required to diagnose humeral fractures. As with any shoulder injury, these children should be assessed with a complete three-view shoulder series: an anterior-posterior view of the glenohumeral joint (rather than the torso), an axillary view, and a scapular Y view. The last two views are necessary to assess the glenohumeral relationship properly and to rule out any dislocation or subluxation.

Classification

Metaphyseal proximal humeral fractures are classified by their anatomic location, displacement, and angulation. Proximal humerus physeal fractures are commonly diagnosed according to the Salter Harris classification scheme. Most of these fractures are either nondisplaced Salter Harris I fractures, or displaced Salter Harris II fractures. It is extremely rare to see a Salter Harris III or IV proximal humerus fracture. Neer and Horwitz [9] classified pediatric proximal humerus fractures based on the amount of displacement. Grade I fractures had less than 5 mm of displacement; grade II had between 5 mm and one third the diameter of the humeral shaft; grade III had between one third and two thirds the diameter of the humeral shaft; and grade III fractures had displacement greater than two thirds the diameter of the humeral shaft. The Neer classification scheme is rarely used clinically today.

Treatment

Because of their tremendous healing and remodeling potential, most proximal humerus fractures in children should be treated nonoperatively. This treatment has been the traditional one, regardless of age or displacement. More recently, some favorable reports have been published suggesting that, in older children with marked displacement, operative treatment should be considered [10,11].

For the truly nondisplaced or minimally displaced fracture, treatment in a sling or shoulder immobilizer is all that is necessary. For infants, a sling and swath (with the arm wrapped to the torso by an Ace wrap) is sufficient. Parents are instructed in the skin care of the infant, and in the reapplication of the swath. Because of the early healing potential and the massive callous that is typically formed, only 4 weeks of immobilization are required.

Either sling immobilization or a shoulder immobilizer should be used for minimally displaced proximal humerus fractures. Gentle pendulum exercises should be started between 2 and 4 weeks, and active range of motion should be started between 4 and 6 weeks. Most patients can resume overhead activities by that point, and should expect normal or near-normal function 2 months from the date of injury.

Most pediatric orthopedic surgeons would agree that even markedly displaced fractures in children younger than 10 should be treated nonoperatively. In this young patient population, the massive remodeling potential of the proximal humerus will allow even the most displaced fracture to heal and eventually remodel to a normal-appearing, fully functional shoulder [12,13].

The actual indications for closed reduction or operative treatment are controversial. The literature contains no generally accepted guidelines for acceptable angulation and displacement. Beringer and colleagues [13] reported on 48 patients who had displaced proximal humerus fractures. Nine children were treated operatively, and one had complications. They examined the functional results of those patients who had "acceptable" displacement and those patients who had a radiographic malunion; neither group had functional deficits.

Many centers treat patients who have significantly displaced fractures with an attempt at closed reduction, usually in the operating room with anesthesia [13]. The technique of closed reduction involves traction, abduction, forward flexion, and external rotation of the arm. If the fracture is unstable, percutaneous fixation with smooth K-wires is the preferred fixation method [14]. The patients treated with a successful closed reduction are immobilized for 4 to 6 weeks, followed by active range of motion. If pins are used, they are routinely removed at 3 to 4 weeks.

Open treatment is reserved for those patients who have displaced intra-articular fractures or those with neurovascular compromise, which is extremely rare in the pediatric patient population. The open approach is typically through a delto-pectoral approach. Humeral head fractures should be treated with countersunk cancellous screws.

Complications

Complications are rare in the treatment of proximal humerus fractures in children. For neonatal fractures, concomitant brachial plexus palsy may occur, and the clinician should be alert to this possibility [15]. The infants should be followed with serial neurologic examinations to rule out this severe injury. The most common complication of proximal humerus fractures is a mild shortening of the humerus, which may occur more frequently in older children [9]. However, this upper extremity limb length inequality rarely causes any functional disability, and often is not clinically apparent. Varus radiographic malunion is also a reported complication, but again, it rarely causes any functional limitation [16]. Neurovascular injury with proximal humerus fractures is rare in the pediatric population.

Fractures of the humeral shaft

Like proximal humerus fractures, fractures of the humeral shaft are rare in children, representing fewer than 10% of all humerus fractures in children [17]. Also like proximal humerus fractures, humeral diaphyseal fractures in children are often treated without surgical intervention. Humeral shaft fractures are most often seen in neonates, and this fracture is the second most common birth fracture, behind clavicle fractures. Neonatal humeral shaft fractures have a reported prevalence ranging from 0.035% to 0.35% [18].

History and physical examination

The mechanism of injury can be similar to that of proximal humerus fractures, and can be a simple fall on an outstretched hand or a direct blow to the upper extremity. Fractures of the humeral shaft are often either transverse fractures or spiral fractures. Humeral shaft fractures in adolescents commonly occur during sporting activities. Humeral shaft fractures also occur in relatively high-energy trauma, such as in a motor vehicle collision. Again, fractures that occur with minimal history of trauma should alert the physician to a possible pathologic fracture, such as a simple bone cyst or in the setting of fibrous dysplasia [7].

Humeral shaft fractures can occur with birth trauma, and are more common with large infants and breech presentation. Also, like proximal humerus fractures, pediatric humeral shaft fractures can occur in the setting of child abuse or nonaccidental trauma.

Patients present complaining of pain and swelling in the midaspect of the arm. The infant presents with the observation by the parent, pediatrician, or nurses that the child will not move the upper extremity. Occasionally, a deformity is obvious, but most fractures are relatively minimally displaced and do not usually have significant deformities. The fracture usually occurs distal to the deltoid insertion, and the rotator cuff muscles and deltoid muscles displace the proximal fragment anteriorly and laterally, in abduction. Usually, the distal fragment is shortened and has medial displacement from the pull of the biceps and triceps. The distal fragment is usually rotated internally because of the position of the arm, which is usually held across the chest to minimize motion and pain. As in all fractures, a thorough, detailed neurovascular examination is essential. As in adult humeral shaft fractures, these fractures in children can be associated with a radial nerve injury.

Imaging

The imaging of humeral shaft fractures in children is very straightforward. In most cases, anterior-posterior and lateral views of the humerus are sufficient. As in every fracture in orthopedics, the joint above and the joint below the fracture should also be adequately visualized. If these joints are not well seen on the humerus view, then dedicated shoulder and elbow series should be obtained.

Classification

Classification of pediatric humeral diaphyseal fractures is often descriptive, classifying the fracture based on location, fracture pattern (spiral, transverse, and so forth), displacement, and angulation. The Association for the Study of Internal Fixation (AO-ASIF) has a classification system for humeral shaft fractures, but its usefulness in pediatric fractures is limited [19].

Treatment

Regardless of the fracture displacement, obstetric fractures in neonates are treated with simple immobilization, with a swath holding the infant's arms to the chest for 3 to 4 weeks. The parents should be taught how to apply this bandage and how to provide bathing care for the child for these first few weeks. These very young children will heal these fractures very quickly and with abundant callous formation in a very short time. Parents should also be warned of the palpable callous mass that will form. Furthermore, the parents should be reassured about the powerful remodeling potential of these fractures, and that, even when they are completely displaced and severely angulated, the child will heal and remodel the fracture, and should go on to have a fully functional upper extremity. However, these children should be followed well past the healing of the fracture to assess brachial plexus function, to assure that a concomitant nerve injury does not exist [3].

Most minimally to moderately displaced pediatric humeral shaft fractures are also treated with closed treatment. In all ages, angulation of less than 20° to 30° is well tolerated, and varus malalignment of more than 30° is necessary before becoming clinically apparent. Beaty [20] described acceptable displacements and angulation with an age-based algorithm: for children under 5, 70° of angulation and total displacement; for children 5 to 12, 40° to 70° of angulation; and, for children older than 12, 40° of angulation and 50% apposition. In younger children, bayonet apposition is acceptable, and shortening of 1 to 2 centimeters is well tolerated. Clinical deformity (or lack thereof) is more important than radiographic alignment.

Initially, the child is placed in a coaptation splint for approximately 2 weeks. If the fracture is truly minimally displaced, the child is then placed in a Sarmiento-type clamshell brace for another 4 weeks, or until adequate callous formation is seen [21]. For fractures that have acceptable angulation but have some shortening, the child can be treated in a hanging arm cast until adequate healing is seen. Shoulder range-of-motion exercises are typically started 4 weeks after the original date of injury.

Operative treatment of pediatric humeral shaft fractures is usually performed only in the setting of open fractures or in those rare cases in closed fractures when acceptable displacement or angulation cannot be improved and controlled with closed means. External fixation techniques have been described for those cases with severe soft tissue loss [22]. External fixators are also useful in the setting of severe bone loss, where distraction osteogenesis may be the preferred mode of reconstruction. Flexible titanium nails are an excellent choice for internal fixation for open fractures and for fractures in polytrauma patients [23]. Open reduction internal fixation with plating techniques is generally reserved for open fractures.

Complications

The two most common complications of humeral shaft fractures in adults are rare in children: radial nerve palsy and nonunion. Complete nerve injury is rare in closed fractures in children, and nerve function usually recovers spontaneously [24]. A radial nerve palsy in the setting of a closed humeral shaft fracture in a child should not be treated with open reduction and exploration of the nerve. These patients should have a proactive conservative treatment strategy, with wrist splints and physical therapy to maintain a full range of motion and prevent wrist contractures. If the patient still has no evidence of recovery after 3 months, he/she should be evaluated with electromyogram and nerve conduction velocity studies.

Nonunion of the humeral shaft is extremely uncommon in pediatric patients, and has been reported rarely in the literature [25]. Delayed union can often be treated successfully with ultrasound bone stimulation. Radiographic description of the healed humeral shaft fracture should not be called a malunion, unless the angulation is more than 30°. Like proximal humerus fractures, neurovascular injuries resulting from humeral diaphyseal fractures are rare in children.

References

[1] Mizuta T, Benson WM, Foster BK, et al. Statistical analysis of the incidence of physeal injuries. J Pediatr Orthop 1987;7:518–23.

[2] Landin LA. Epidemiology of children's fractures. J Pediatr Orthop 1997;6:79–83.

[3] Shulman BH, Terhune CB. Epiphyseal injuries in breech delivery. Pediatrics 1951;8:693–700.

[4] Beaty JH, Kasser JR. Rockwood and Wilkins' fractures in children. 5th edition. Philadelphia: Lippincott Williams and Wilkins; 2001. p. 741–806.

[5] Nordqvist A, Petersson CJ. Incidence and causes of shoulder girdle injuries in an urban population. J Shoulder Elbow Surg 1995;4:107–12.

[6] Jeffrey CC. Fracture separation of the upper humeral epiphysis. Surg Gynecol Obstet 1953;96:205–9.
[7] Ahn JI, Park JS. Pathological fractures secondary to unicameral bone cysts. Int Orthop 1994;18:20–2.
[8] Kohler R, Trillaud JM. Fracture and fracture separation of the proximal humerus in children: a report of 136 cases. J Pediatr Orthop 1983;202:1–xx.
[9] Neer CS III, Horwitz BS. Fractures of the proximal humeral epiphyseal plate. Clin Orthop 1965;41:24–xx.
[10] Markel DC, Donley BG, Blasier RB. Percutaneous intramedullary pinning of proximal humeral fractures. Orthop Rev 1994;23:667–71.
[11] Bishop JY, Flatow EL. Pediatric shoulder trauma. Clin Orthop Relat Res 2005;432:41–8.
[12] Dameron TB Jr, Reibel DB. Fractures involving the proximal humeral epiphyseal plate. J Bone Joint Surg Am 1969;51:289–97.
[13] Beringer DC, Weiner DS, Nobel JS, et al. Severely displaced proximal humerus epiphyseal fractures: a follow-up study. J Pediatr Orthop 1998;18:31–xx.
[14] Naidu SH, Bixler B, Capo JT, et al. Percuataneous pinning of proximal humerus fractures: a biomechanical study. Orthopedics 1997;20:1073–xx.
[15] Drew SJ, Giddins GE, Birch R. A slowly evolving brachial plexus injury following a proximal humerus fractures in a child. J Hand Surg 1995;20:24–5.
[16] Ellefsen BK, Frierson MA, Raney EM, et al. Humerus varus: a complication of neonatal, infantile, and childhood injury and infection. J Pediatr Orthop 1994;14:479–86.
[17] Cheng JC, Shen WY. Limb fracture pattern in different pediatric age groups: a study of 3350 children. J Orthop Trauma 1993;7:15–22.
[18] Madsen TE. Fractures of the extremities in the newborn. Acta Obstet Gynecol Scand 1955;34:4.
[19] Muller ME, Allgower M, Schneider R, et al. Manual of internal fixation. Techniques recommended by the AO-ASIF group. 3rd edition. Berlin: Springer-Verlag; 1991.
[20] Beaty JH. Fractures of the proximal humerus and shaft in children. Instr Course Lect 1992;41:369–72.
[21] Sarmiento A, Horowitch A, Aboulafia A, et al. Functional bracing for comminuted extra-articular fractures of the distal third of the humerus. J Bone Joint Surg Br 1990;72:283–7.
[22] Asche G. Use of external fixation in pediatric fractures. Zentralbl Chir 1986;111:391–7.
[23] Huber RI, Keller HW, Huber PM, et al. Flexible intramedullary nailing as fracture treatment in children. J Pediatr Orthop 1996;16:602–5.
[24] Shah JJ, Bhatti NA. Radial nerve paralysis associated with fractures of the humerus: a review of 62 cases. Clin Orthop 1983;172:171–xx.
[25] Lewallen RP, Peterson HA. Nonunion of long bone fractures in children: a review of 30 cases. J Pediatr Orthop 1985;5:135–xx.

ELSEVIER
SAUNDERS

Hand Clin 23 (2007) 437–448

HAND
CLINICS

The Operative Treatment of Diaphyseal Humeral Shaft Fractures

Peter A. Cole, MD[a,*], Coen A. Wijdicks, MSc[b]

[a]*Department of Orthopaedic Surgery, University of Minnesota, Regions Hospital, 640 Jackson Street, Saint Paul, MN 55101, USA*

[b]*Department of Orthopaedic Surgery, University of Minnesota, 2512 South Seventh Street, R200, Minneapolis, MN 55454, USA*

Fractures of the humeral shaft comprise 1% to 3% of all fractures [1–4]. Incidence rates reveal a bimodal distribution in which there is one small peak during adolescence, followed by a larger spike during the fifth and sixth decades of life [3]. Most humeral diaphysis fractures are simple patterns of the mid-diaphysis. Beginning in the sixth decade, women are more prone to humeral shaft fractures. It is helpful to consider two classes of injuries when considering operative management of this fracture, those which occur in good quality bone, and those that fall into the class of fragility fractures. Different techniques and thought processes may come to play for each category, as well as for those fractures that may be classified as high-energy injuries (with multifragmentation and large displacement) versus low-energy injuries (characterized by simple fracture patterns).

There has been a significant evolution of thought and practice with regard to the treatment of humeral shaft fractures. Although surgical techniques have become popularized over the past couple of decades, conservative management has played an important role historically and continues to be the mainstay of treatment. There have been alternating operative trends emphasizing different types of plating and nailing techniques. Both plate and intramedullary fixation each have been popularized and have their respective proponents. More recently, there seems to be slightly more enthusiasm for plating largely based on the commonly encountered outcome of shoulder pain after antegrade nailing of humerus fractures which is manifest months and years after surgery in a large proportion of patients. Very recently, minimally invasive techniques for plating have been investigated specifically for feasibility and safety, and these newer techniques are finding their way into the treatment armamentarium of some orthopaedic traumatologists.

It has often been said that the general patient population, as well as the contemporary surgical community of orthopedic surgeons, seems to be less tolerant of the more labor-intensive methods of conservative management, less tolerant of what was formerly thought to be acceptable deformity, and less patient with regard to rehabilitation of these injuries. With these trends as a backrop, many relative indications for humerus fracture surgery have emerged, including open humeral shaft fractures, fractures associated with certain radial nerve lesions, floating elbow injuries, polytraumatized patients, and patients with large breasts in whom varus deformity with closed management is commonplace. Even certain fracture patterns such as segmental injuries, as well as proximal and distal third fractures are thought by some to be problematic with functional bracing.

This article emphasizes surgical technique, providing a review of the surgical spectrum of treatment inclusive of intramedullary nailing and plating. However, conservative management of the isolated humeral diaphysis fracture remains an effective treatment; thus, the article begins with a brief discussion of this modality.

* Corresponding author.
E-mail address: peter.a.cole@healthpartners.com (P.A. Cole).

0749-0712/07/$ - see front matter. Published by Elsevier Inc.
doi:10.1016/j.hcl.2007.11.004

Nonoperative treatment

Traditional treatment for most humeral shaft fractures has historically been nonoperative for the majority of closed diaphyseal injuries. High union and satisfaction rates have been published in relatively large series by Sarmiento and colleagues who championed the use of functional bracing for these injuries [5–7]. The union rate of 97% in a series of 620 patients supported the recommendations that are used today for conservative treatment [8–10]. Other studies, however, have determined that the incidence of nonunion after nonoperative treatment is higher for certain fracture patterns and open fractures [8,11,12]. One drawback to functional bracing is the limitation to external rotation in 30% of patients, flexion in 15% of patients, and abduction in 10% of patients. Additionally, elbow flexion and extension are impaired in approximately 8% of patients [6].

The results of two retrospective studies published this past year appear to favor nonoperative management and draw similar conclusions. Both studies employed functional brace treatment of humeral diaphysis fractures until fracture healing, and both reported a nonunion rate of 10% [1,13].

In the Swedish study, which included 78 patients, a trend toward more frequent nonunion in simple fractures was demonstrated (Orthopedic Trauma Association Type A) ($P = .08$), occurring in 18% (7/39) of patients. Fifty of these patients completed long-term outcome examinations, and 50% of the patients reported full recovery after nonoperative treatment. However, none of the patients with a healed nonunion had full recovery after revision surgery ($P < .05$). The authors warn of the simple fracture pattern in the proximal and middle third of the humerus, as a possible indication for surgery due to a higher rate of nonunion [1].

In the Boston study from the Massachusetts General Hospital, the main risk factor was the proximal 1/3 fracture of which 14/49 (29%) of fractures failed to heal; all of which were proximal 1/3 fractures of the long spiral oblique variety. There was no more than 15-degree loss of shoulder or elbow motion in 95% of patients who healed their fracture. It is notable that angular deformity of >20 degrees of varus occurred in three patients, but was not thought to cause functional deformity in either [13].

Extending the theme of the previous two studies, 40/51 consecutive patients available for follow-up with a closed, extra-articular fracture of the distal third of the humeral diaphysis were followed for at least 6 months after either functional bracing or plate fixation [14]. In the operatively treated patients, there was one loss of fixation and one infection. There were three iatrogenic radial nerve palsies, one of which did not resolve by 3 months after surgery. All operatively treated fractures healed with <10° of angular deformity, and only one patient lost 20° of shoulder or elbow motion. Among the nonoperatively treated fractures, two were converted to plate fixation because of concern for alignment, leaving only one patient with >30° of malalignment in any plane. Two patients lost >20° of elbow or shoulder motion, and two patients had development of skin breakdown during brace treatment, leaving the authors to conclude merely that there are pros and cons of both treatment methodologies [14].

Because the shoulder has universal motion with an exceptional physiologic range of motion in many planes, deformity is well tolerated after union (Fig. 1). Klenerman [15] established criteria for acceptance of fracture reduction, which is a guide to conservative management. These criteria include 20° anteroposterior angulation (sagittal plane), 30° varus angulation, or 15° malrotation and 3 cm shortening. Overall, functional bracing seems to provide satisfactory results; however, surgery has a place in the contemporary treatment of these fractures.

Operative management

Indications for surgery

Surgery is indicated for instances in which a closed reduction cannot be maintained. This situation can occur when there is soft tissue interposition (ie, muscle or nerve), extrinsic deforming forces (a large breast), or a significant deformity from muscular forces particularly common in the proximal and distal diaphysis. Rotational deformity is typically well tolerated assuming normal shoulder function. An open fracture, although rare, is an indication for internal fixation, whether by plating or nailing, largely because the surgeon already has access to the surgical site and can effect a more predictable treatment course. Instances of associated articular elbow and shoulder fractures are recommended for open reduction and internal fixation, as is the condition of a floating elbow. Surgical treatment in such combination injuries greatly facilitates rehabilitation, and promotes motion which aids in prevention of a joint contracture.

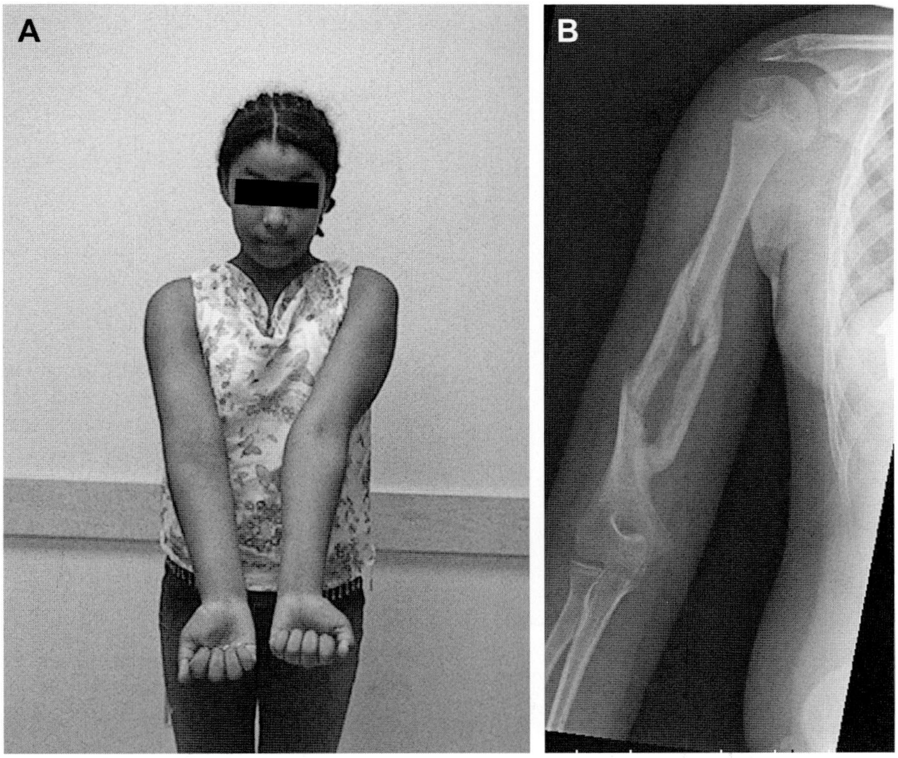

Fig. 1. (*A*) A 14-year-old girl whose parents refused to allow her to have a proposed operation to place an external fixator on the right arm to realign a humeral fracture. She describes her function, motion, and strength to be normal 6 months after the injury, and is not aware of the cosmetic deformity caused by the loss of her carrying angle. (*B*) Anteroposterior view of a humerus 10 weeks after the segmental fracture. Note the healing that has occurred, and the 15-degree varus angular deformity in the coronal plane.

There is controversy over when to surgically intervene in the setting of a nerve injury. The incidence of radial nerve palsy associated with humeral shaft fractures is reported to be between 2% and 17% [16–19]. Most experts currently recommend that any prereduction palsy be managed nonoperatively because the vast majority of such lesions resolve spontaneously. If such a lesion is dense and persistent beyond 6 weeks, then electromyography and nerve conduction studies are warranted to define a baseline examination and the extent of the lesion. Immediate surgical exploration is indicated for instances in which a radial nerve injury is associated with an open fracture, penetrating injury mechanism, or vascular injury (Fig. 2A, B). If a radial nerve examination was noted to be intact before a reduction maneuver was employed, but indicates a deficit after reduction, then urgent exploration is indicated as well. The controversy with regard to immediate versus delayed exploration of an injured radial nerve lies in the fact that subsequent callus formation can potentially encase the radial nerve and make surgical exploration more technically demanding.

In the setting of an impending pathologic humerus fracture, surgery is indicated as well for palliative treatment, and the most appropriate treatment in this clinical scenario is an intramedullary nail, which is used to stabilize the entire bone to protect it from further lesions that could manifest later in the same humerus. Furthermore, a nail will eliminate the need to expose the lesion and also limit blood loss [19–22].

Another common indication for surgery is polytrauma including lower limb fractures that require early crutch mobilization. Rigid internal fixation will offer substantial advantages to overall rehabilitation under these circumstances.

Nailing or plating

There are few Level I evidence studies that have compared the results of plating versus nailing. In 2000, Chapman [23] prospectively

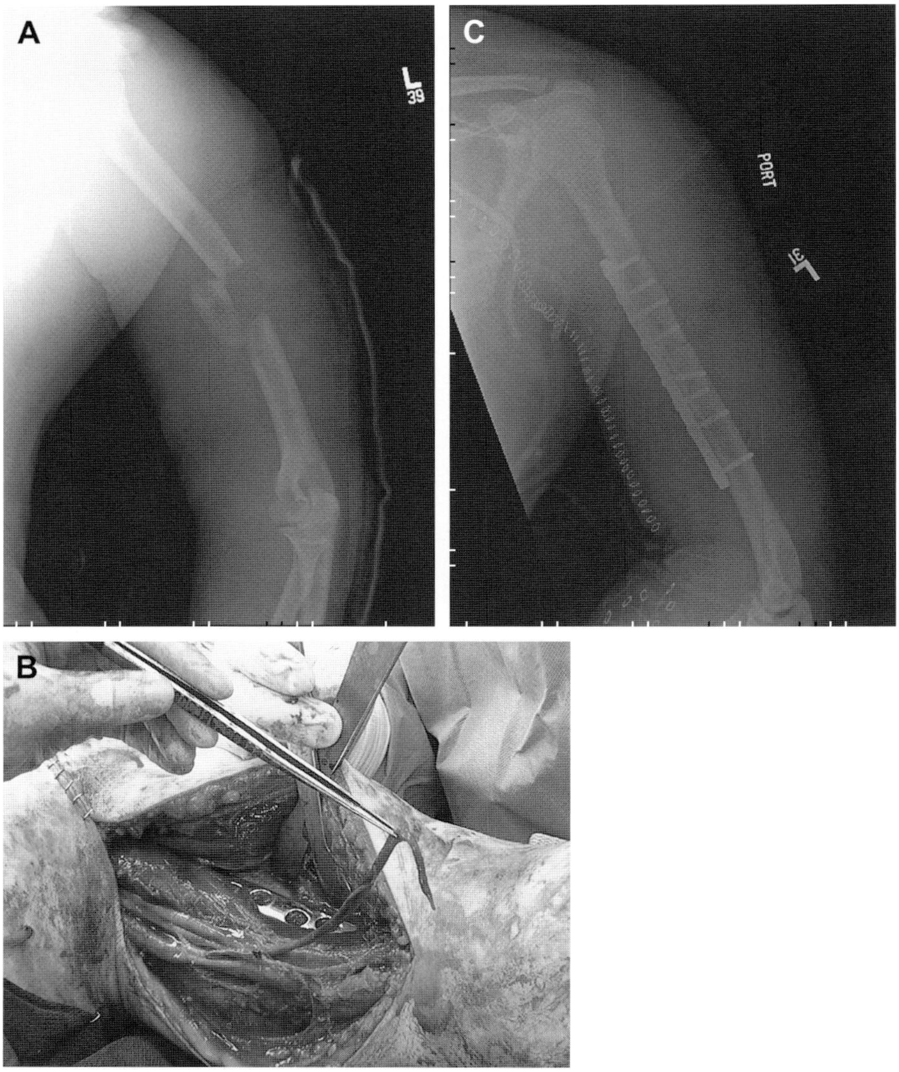

Fig. 2. (*A*) Lateral radiograph of a high-energy humeral fracture sustained after a patient struck a tree on his snowmobile. The segmental bone fragment was 4.5 cm, and the patient presented with a neurologic deficit of the ulnar nerve and traumatic brachial artery pseudoaneurysm. (*B*) Intraoperative photograph of the same patient showing the transected ulnar nerve, which required emergent exploration and was in turn associated with a preoperative polyneurologic deficit. (*C*) Lateral postoperative radiograph shows how the medial approach used for the vascular repair, allowed for anterior placement of a large fragment 4.5-mm broad plate. Direct reduction and interfragmentary compression permits stable fixation, which allows immediate rehabilitation including weight-bearing or lifting activities.

compared antegrade nailing with plating. Nonunion was rare in both treatment groups. Shoulder impingement was the primary complaint occurring in 16% of patients undergoing a nail at a mean follow-up of 13 months. McCormack and colleagues [19] compared plating with antegrade and retrograde nailing. These authors reported a nonunion rate of 4% for plated fractures and 10% for fractures undergoing an intramedullary nailing. In addition, complications were also more significant for the nailing group when compared with the plating group (62% versus 13%). McCormack also found no shoulder impingement or radial nerve palsy in the plating group, and this was not the case for the nailing group in which 31% had shoulder impingement and 14% had radial nerve palsy at final follow-up of 14.3 months. Additional surgery was also required in 33% of the nailing group. In previous reports on plate fixation, nonunion has ranged from 2% to 10%, infection from 2% to 4%, and iatrogenic radial nerve palsy from 0% to 5% [16–19]. Intramedullary nailing studies have reported incidences of nonunion ranging from 0% to 8%, with slightly lower rates for retrograde nailing [20–22,24,25].

Surgical techniques

Plate osteosynthesis

Considering the role of plate fixation for humeral shaft fractures, there are several considerations with regard to the choice of implants. Generally speaking, large fragment implants are preferred for humeral shaft fractures. Traditional AO plating techniques describe the use of a 4.5-mm dynamic compression plate. This implant offers a very strong construct that may be optimal for direct fracture reduction, interfragmentary compression, and primary bone healing.

Although broad 4.5-mm plates have been recommended traditionally, it would seem that such a large and durable implant is likely not necessary given the adherence to current biologic principles of fixation. This point seems particularly true for smaller patients. Most surgeons today prefer 4.5-mm narrow fragment plates used with large fragment screws. Recent advances in plate technology have introduced precontoured plates for periarticular fractures, and to this discussion these would be germane for the more proximal or more distal diaphysial fracture. These plates taper or contour to fit the osseous anatomy and allow for improved fixation enhancement around joints. Another technologic advancement has included the entry of locked plates or fixators in which the screwheads actually lock into the holes of the plate. Locked plates may represent a treatment enhancement in the setting of highly comminuted or segmental fractures, or in the setting of osteoporosis where failure after cyclic bending or torsional forces have higher thresholds than conventional plate and screw constructs.

Though track records for conventional plate and screw fixation reveal exceptional results with regard to fracture union, such series generally have not included high proportions of osteoporotic patients or complex injury variants in which these newer technologies may improve or optimize results. Furthermore, it is possible that these stronger mechanical solutions may allow for shorter plates, smaller incisions, or perhaps earlier and more aggressive rehabilitation.

There have been many approaches described concerning the open reduction and internal fixation of the humerus. Humeral diaphyseal plating may be accomplished through either an extended lateral approach, anterolateral, posterior, or medial approach [26–29]. The extended lateral approach exposes the intermuscular plane between the triceps and the anterior compartment musculature. The patient should be positioned supine for this approach, which is ideal for the distal two thirds of the humerus and also takes advantage of an exposure of the radial nerve [29]. The anterior approach is primarily used in proximal and middle third fractures. Proximally, the deltopectoral interval is used, whereas the distal incision develops the lateral border of the biceps musculature. Very distal in this approach, the radial nerve will be visualized lying between the brachialis and brachioradialis. The posterior approach may be the most popular approach, though it is best used for distal third humeral fractures, where it provides exposure to the humerus through the interval between the lateral and long ends of the triceps muscle [29]. The posterior approach will also locate the radial nerve as it courses along the lateral border of the medial head of the triceps just after leaving he spiral groove [30,31]. The medial approach to the humeral shaft exposes the insertion of the pectoralis major muscle proximally down to the coronoid fossa distally [27]. This approach develops the interval between the biceps and triceps musculature,

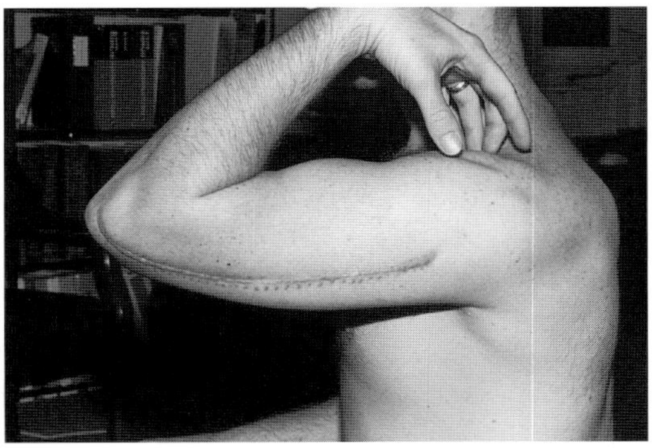

Fig. 3. This patient, who sustained a segmental humerus shaft fracture a year earlier, had a good functional outcome; however, some patients regard this type of scar as unsightly, making it a drawback to this method of treatment.

and requires exposure and protection of the ulnar nerve and brachial artery.

Because the advantages of traditional plate fixation have been described with its associated modest rate of complications, the unsightly scar is not often mentioned in the list of drawbacks to this procedure (Fig. 3). The posterior and certainly the medial approach are less conspicuous and should be considered if vanity weighs heavily in the patient's consideration for surgery (Fig. 4).

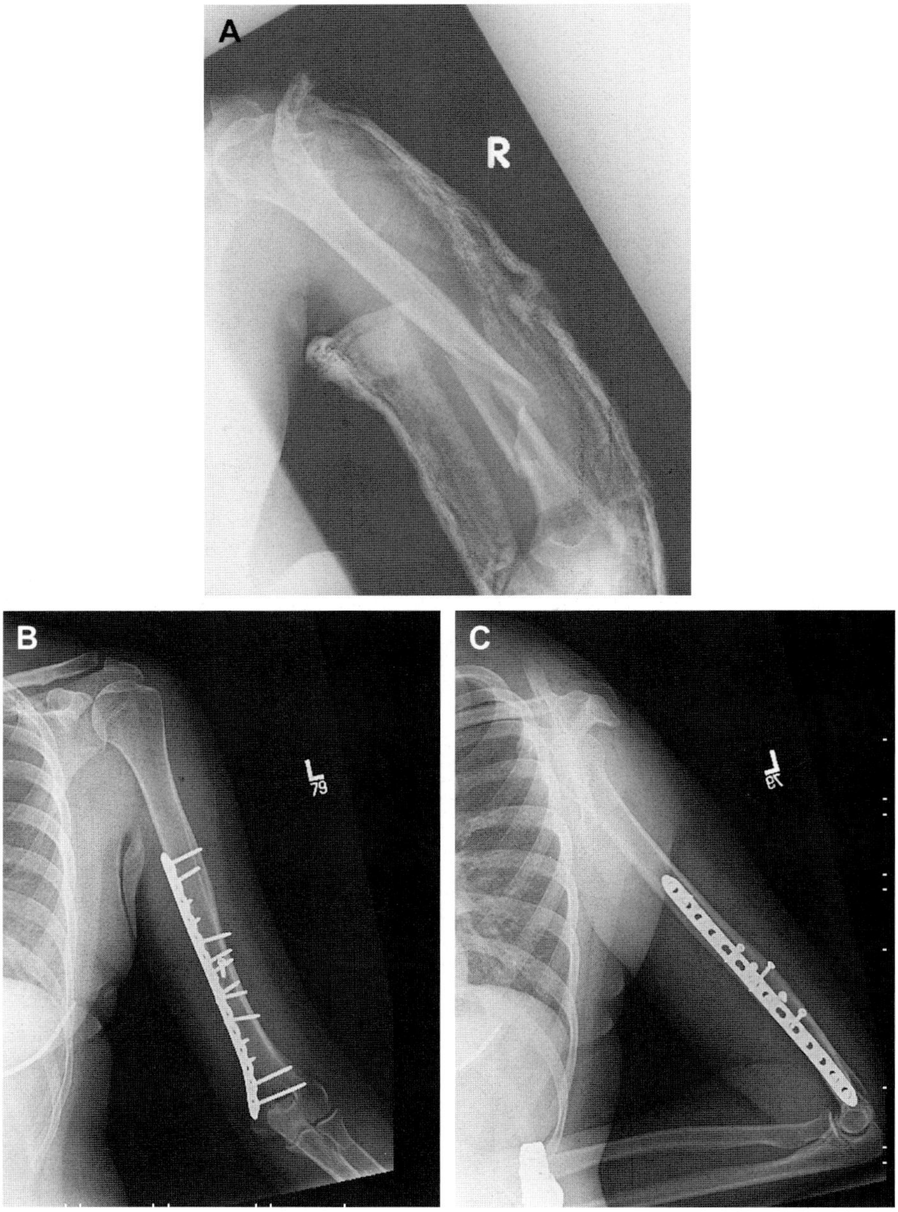

Fig. 4. (*A*) Anteroposterior radiograph of a patient who presented with a closed humeral fracture treated with a coaptation splint and an ankle fracture after crashing her bicycle. The patient wanted to get back to work as soon as possible, and required the use of her left arm for crutches which was allowed as soon as her pain subsided. She appreciated the idea of having a scar concealed toward the inside of her arm, which is what the medial approach required. (*B*) Anteroposterior radioigraph of the humerus after healing. (*C*) Lateral radiograph of the humerus after healing. The patient eventually requested that her plate be removed due to irritation above the medial epicondyle.

Furthermore, plate fixation allows for exploration of the radial nerve, which may be beneficial, though a miniopen approach can always be added to the surgical tactic of a nailing procedure if there is a concern of nerve entrapment.

Intramedullary nailing

The use of intramedullary nailing may provide a biomechanical advantage during early weight-bearing, depending on the fracture pattern, because the nail is considered a load-sharing device. Though original nailing techniques employed the use of multiple flexible nails, more recent use of interlocking intramedullary implants has become fairly standard practice. Despite the attractiveness of a smaller approach, intramedullary nailing techniques in general have yielded nonunion rates of up to 30%, indicating that

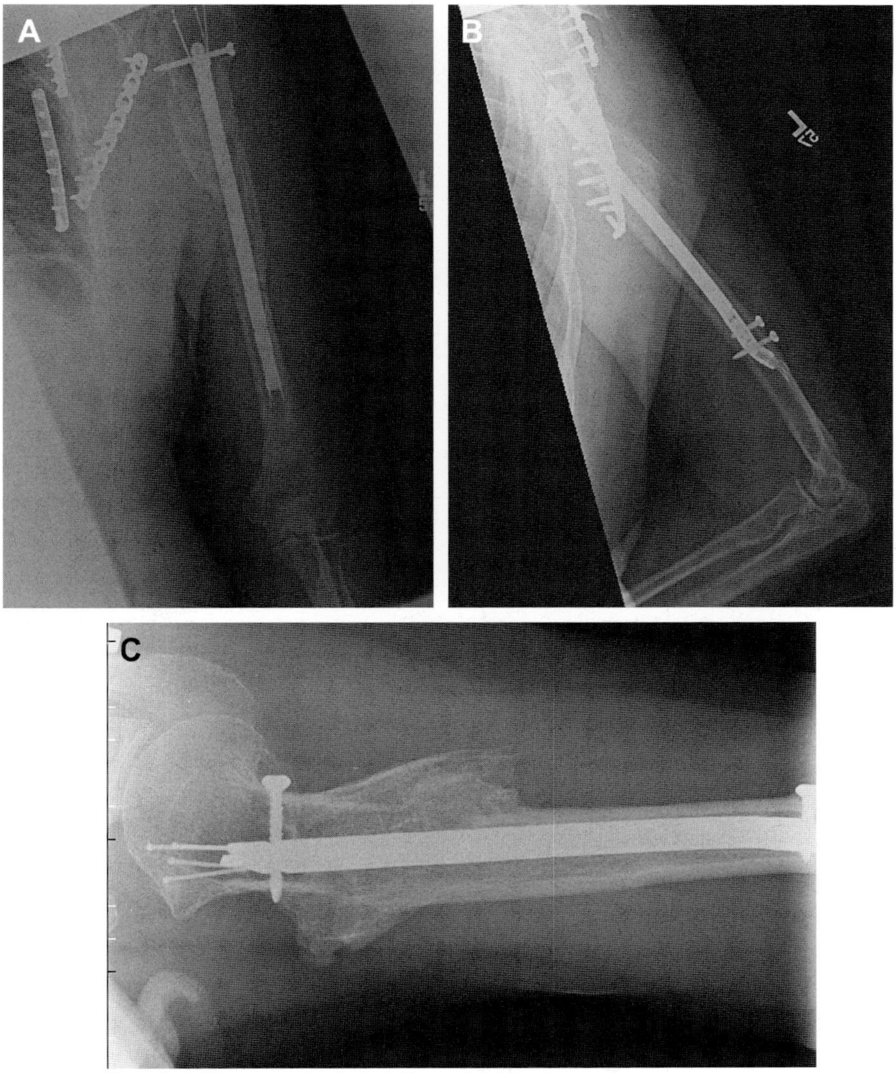

Fig. 5. (*A*) Anteroposterior view of a humerus after treatment and healing. The fracture was fixed with a retrograde flexible locking nail. A retrograde approach was used to avoid superimposing shoulder pain or stiffness associated with an antegrade nailing, because this patient had an ipsilateral displaced glenoid neck fracture. (*B*) Lateral view of the humerus shows the static locking, posterior starting point in the distal humerus, and successful fracture union. Because the posterior approach for the scapula required the lateral decubitus position, the retrograde humeral nail was able to be inserted during the same operative session. (*C*) An axillary view of the shoulder showing the humeral shaft healed with robust callus, but in 5° of fracture flexion that was well tolerated by the patient.

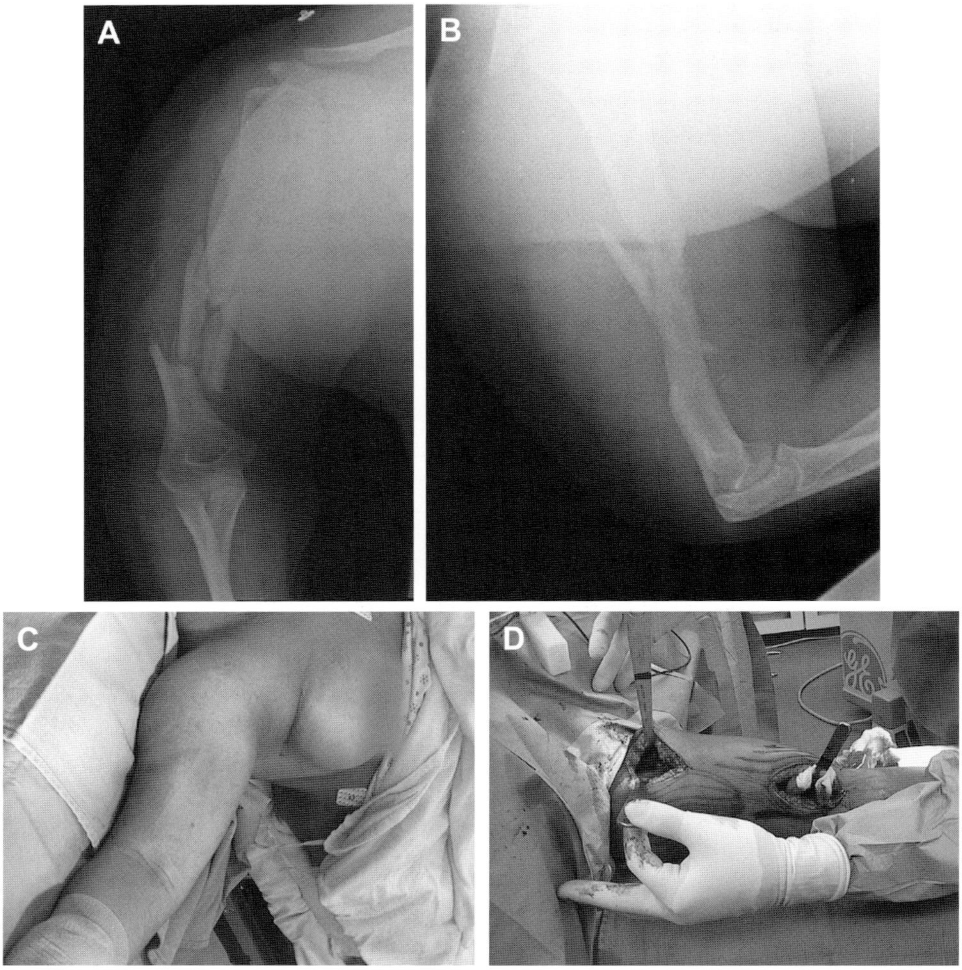

Fig. 6. (*A*) Anteroposterior radiograph of a segmental humeral fracture sustained after a fall in a very obese woman. (*B*) Lateral radiograph of the humerus in the same patient. (*C*) Intraoperative positioning for a minimally invasive plating procedure, allowing an appreciation of the rationale for operative treatment, specifically that her anatomy caused the fracture to fall into varus with attempt at closed management with a coaptation splint. (*D*) Intraoperative photograph shows the approach used proximally and distally to fix the fracture. In the distal wound, the radial nerve was identified and protected. (*E*) Intraoperative fluoroscopic image depicting alignment of the fracture on a lateral. No direct reduction of the fracture was performed. (*F*) Intraoperative fluoroscopy shot depicting alignment of the fracture on an anteroposterior view. Distal fixation with locking screws was obtained, and alignment appeared to be satisfactory. (*G*) Postoperative lateral radiograph shows good sagittal plane alignment. (*H*) Postoperative anteroposterior radiograph shows much more varus then was suspected intraoperatively. Though this was not clinically significant, it underscores the challenge of obtaining a good reduction using minimally invasive surgery.

excellent surgical technique and patient selection is paramount. One study by Riemer and colleagues [32] examined 40 fractures of the humeral diaphysis treated with 9-mm-diameter Seidel nails. This study reported a 58% complication rate (comminution, infection, nonunion) when compared with the larger diameter canal of 10 mm, which reported only a 4% complication rate [32]. Additionally, the radial nerve is at a direct risk with closed reduction and canal preparation. With this technique, it is also not possible to free an entrapped radial nerve from the fracture. If an intramedullary nailing procedure is planned in cases where radial nerve palsy is present before surgery, or in the cases in which a neurologic examination cannot be performed in an awake

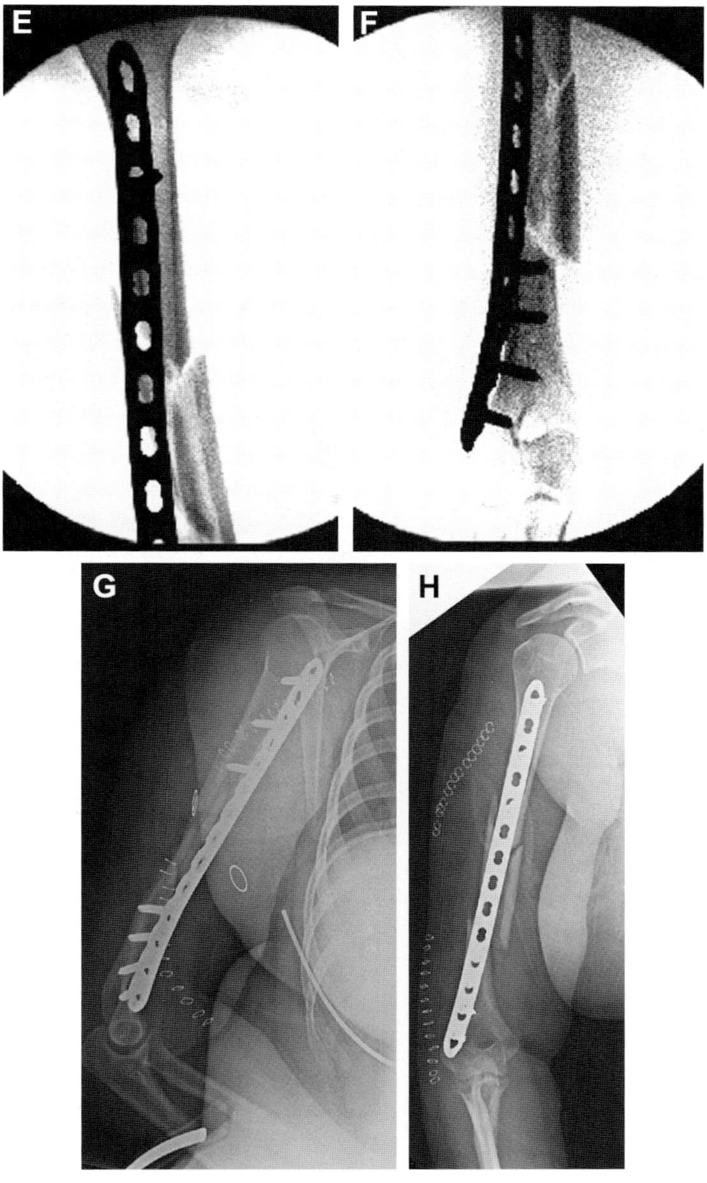

Fig. 6 (*continued*)

patient, then the procedure should be combined with a miniopen approach to the fracture to insure that the nerve is cleared.

Antegrade intramedullary nailing

Antegrade intramedullary nails are performed through a small deltoid splitting incision off the lateral edge of the acromion, making a careful inicision through the rotator cuff, before preparing the entry with an awl or guide wire. The drawback to this technique is the fact that the entry requires access through the rotator cuff, which may be the culprit in shoulder pain [23]. However, Flinkkila and colleagues [33] found no statistical difference in shoulder pain, functional scores, or isometric strength parameters between uncomplicated cases of antegrade intramedullary nailing and dynamic compression plating. They concluded that other factors are responsible for shoulder joint impairment and need to be investigated further. It is imperative after placing the intramedullary nail that fracture gap is eliminated (perhaps by backslapping the distal fragment) before locking proximally and distally. Because the humerus is not a weight-bearing longbone, fracture gap may explain the variance in rates of nonunion.

There is one antigrade nailing technique that employs the use of a locked flexible nail that can be introduced just distal to the supraspinatous insertion on the greater tuberosity, thus potentially avoiding problems related to shoulder pain. Stannard and colleagues [34] prospectively evaluated 51 humeral shaft fractures using this particular implant. These authors documented a higher complication rate using small-diameter nails consistent with previous literature which highlights increased nonunion and hardware failure rates in patients with small humeral diameters treated with small diameters nails. In this study, it is interesting that though the majority of patients (38 of 42 shoulders) had minimal or no pain, and 36 of 42 patients demonstrated a full range of motion, shoulder pain was not entirely eliminated altogether [34].

Retrograde intramedullary nailing

Retrograde intramedullary nailing consists of inserting nails into the humeral intramedullary canal through an entry porthole just proximal to the olecranon fossa (Fig. 5A, B). This technique minimizes the complications related to shoulder pain seen with antegrade nailing; however, it is associated with its own rate of mild contracture at the elbow joint. Furthermore, though not shown to be a major problem, there is significant stress concentration at the distal nail, which may create a risk for fracture in the supracondylar region of the humerus.

Minimally invasive plate osteosynthesis

Minimally invasive plate osteosynthesis has gained recent attention and has demonstrated satisfactory clinical outcomes in small case series of certain long bones [35–37]. Studies have demonstrated the feasibility of applying this technique in an anterior approach for humeral fractures [37]. There are no clear outcome studies or well-controlled trials on this technique. However, the possible advantages of combining a biologically friendly approach, with strengths of plating (and avoiding the disadvantages of nailing), and a cosmetic advantage, is attractive. On the other hand, given that open plating has yielded strong results with regard to complication rates and union, strong skepticism is appropriate before embracing minimally invasive plating of humerus fractures. Because the surgeon typically obtains a reduction, and executes fixation from anatomic sites remote from the fracture to preserve the biologic milieu surrounding the injury, this technique may be associated with increased rates of malreduction or injury from percutaneous placement of instruments and hardware (Fig. 6A–F).

External fixation

External fixation has played a relatively small role in the treatment of humeral diaphysis fractures; however, it should remain in the armamentarium of the orthopedic surgeon, because it is a good option for patients who present with open mangled extremities or gunshot wounds with segmental comminution and bone loss with associated soft tissue injury. In particular, it is often wise to treat such patients with the provisional stability offered by external fixation while proper debridement and irrigation take place. This provisional method of stabilization is often followed by free tissue transposition when the wounds are stabilized. Eventually, when the soft tissue envelope allows, consideration for conversion to open plating with or without bone grafting would provide a rational course of treatment in these more complex variants. Adequate stability should be achieved with two 4- or 5-mm Schantz pins properly spaced, with a keen understanding of critical neurovascular structures and their locations as they course the brachium. In the danger zones, a small open technique for pin placement is wise to prevent iatrogenic injury to nerves particularly germane distal laterally for the radial nerve and proximal laterally for the axillary nerve.

Summary

Surgical management of humeral shaft fractures has found a broad role in contemporary orthopedic treatment. That being stated, conservative management of the vast majority of humeral shaft fractures will yield satisfactory results with high union rates using short-term splintage followed by functional bracing. Generally speaking, such results come with the acceptance of certain degrees of modest deformity mostly well tolerated by patients. Given the emergence of more indications for surgery, both intramedulary nailing of humeral shaft fractures and plate osteosynthesis have played expanding roles in present-day orthopedic medicine. Such techniques generally have very good track records; however, recognition of important risks and drawbacks is critical for an appropriate presentation of the pros and cons of conservative versus operative management. Today, minimally invasive techniques are being explored to reduce the surgical footprint of the surgeon, while providing an appropriate mechanical solution in the context of an optimal biologic milieu, to promote quickest healing and return to optional function.

References

[1] Ekholm R, Adami J, Tidermark J, et al. Fractures of the shaft of the humerus: an epidemiological study of 401 fractures. J Bone Joint Surg Br 2006;88-B: 1469–73.

[2] Mann RJ, Neal EG. Fractures of the shaft of the humerus in adults. South Med J 1965;58:264–8.

[3] Tytherleigh-Strong G, Walls N, McQueen MM. The epidemiology of humeral shaft fractures. J Bone Joint Surg Br 1998;80:249–53.

[4] Ward EF, Savoie FH, Hughes JL. Fractures of the diaphyseal humerus. In: Skeletal trauma: fractures, dislocations, ligamentous injuries, vol 2. Philadelphia: WB Saunders; 1998. p. 1523–47, Philadelphia.

[5] Balfour GW, Marrero CE. Fracture brace for the treatment of humerus shaft fractures caused by gunshot wounds. Orthop Clin North Am 1995;26: 55–63.

[6] Sarmiento A, Kinman P, Galvin E, et al. Functional bracing of fractures of the shaft of the humerus. J Bone Joint Surg Am 1977;59:596–601.

[7] Wallny T, Westermann K, Sagebiel C, et al. Functional treatment of humeral shaft fractures: indications and results. J Orthop Trauma 1997; 11:283–7.

[8] Sarmiento A, Zagorski JB, Zych GA, et al. Functional bracing for the treatment of fractures of the humeral diaphysis. J Bone Joint Surg Am 2000;82: 478–86.

[9] Koch PP, Gross DF, Gerber C. The results of functional (sarmiento) bracing of humeral shaft fractures. J Shoulder Elbow Surg 2002;11:143–50.

[10] Zagorski J, Latta L, Zych G, et al. Diaphyseal fractures of the humerus. Treatment with prefabricated braces. J Bone Joint Surg Am 1988;70:607–10.

[11] Dameron TB Jr, Grubb SA. Humeral shaft fractures in adults. South Med J 1981;74:1461–7.

[12] Osman N, Touam C, Masmejean E, et al. Results of non-operative and operative treatment of humeral shaft fractures. A series of 104 cases. Chir Main 1998;17:195–206.

[13] Rutgers M, Ring D. Treatment of diaphyseal fractures of the humerus using a functional brace. J Orthop Trauma 2006;20:597–601.

[14] Jawa A, McCarty P, Doornberg J, et al. Extra-articular distal-third diaphyseal fractures of the humerus. A comparison of functional bracing and plate fixation. J Bone Joint Surg Am 2006;88:2343–7.

[15] Klenerman L. Experimental fractures of the adult humerus. Med Biol Eng 1969;7:357–64.

[16] Bell MJ, Beauchamp CG, Kellam JK, et al. The results of plating humeral shaft fractures in patients with multiple injuries. The sunnybrook experience. J Bone Joint Surg Br 1985;67:293–6.

[17] Dabezies EJ, Banta CJ 2nd, Murphy CP, et al. Plate fixation of the humeral shaft for acute fractures, with and without radial nerve injuries. J Orthop Trauma 1992;6:10–3.

[18] Heim D, Herkert F, Hess P, et al. Surgical treatment of humeral shaft fractures–the basel experience. J Trauma 1993;35:226–32.

[19] McCormack RG, Brien D, Buckley RE, et al. Fixation of fractures of the shaft of the humerus by dynamic compression plate or intramedullary nail: a prospective, randomized trial. J Bone Joint Surg Br 2000;82-B:336–9.

[20] Crolla RM, de Vries LS, Clevers GJ. Locked intramedullary nailing of humeral fractures. Injury 1993;24:403–6.

[21] Hems TE, Bhullar TP. Interlocking nailing of humeral shaft fractures: the oxford experience 1991 to 1994. Injury 1996;27:485–9.

[22] Ingman A, Waters D. Locked intramedullary nailing of humeral shaft fractures. implant design, surgical technique, and clinical results. J Bone Joint Surg Br 1994;76-B:23–9.

[23] Chapman JR, Henley MB, Agel J, et al. Randomized prospective study of humeral shaft fracture fixation: intramedullary nails versus plates. J Orthop Trauma 2000;14:162–6.

[24] Robinson C, Bell K, Court-Brown C, et al. Locked nailing of humeral shaft fractures. experience in Edinburgh over a two-year period. J Bone Joint Surg Br 1992;74-B:558–62.

[25] Rommens PM, Blum J, Runkel M. Retrograde nailing of humeral shaft fractures. Clin Orthop Relat Res 1998;(350):26–39.

[26] VanderGriend R, Tomasin J, Ward E. Open reduction and internal fixation of humeral shaft fractures. Results using AO plating techniques. J Bone Joint Surg Am 1986;68:430–3.

[27] Jupiter J. Complex non-union of the humeral diaphysis. Treatment with a medial approach, an anterior plate, and a vascularized fibular graft. J Bone Joint Surg Am 1990;72:701–7.

[28] Bone LB. Fractures of the shaft of the humerus. In: Chapman MW, editor. Operative orthopaedics. edition 2. Philadelphia: JB Lippincott Company; 1993. p. 425–38.

[29] Mills WJ, Hanel DP, Smith DG. Lateral approach to the humeral shaft: an alternative approach for fracture treatment. J Orthop Trauma 1996;10: 81–6.

[30] Uhl RL, Larosa JM, Sibeni T, et al. Posterior approaches to the humerus: when should you worry

about the radial nerve? J Orthop Trauma 1996;10: 338–40.
[31] Gerwin M, Hotchkiss R, Weiland A. Alternative operative exposures of the posterior aspect of the humeral diaphysis with reference to the radial nerve. J Bone Joint Surg Am 1996;78:1690–5.
[32] Riemer BL, Foglesong ME, Burke CJ 3rd, et al. Complications of seidel intramedullary nailing of narrow diameter humeral diaphyseal fractures. Orthopedics 1994;17:19–29.
[33] Flinkkila T, Hyvonen P, Siira P, et al. Recovery of shoulder joint function after humeral shaft fracture: a comparative study between antegrade intramedullary nailing and plate fixation. Arch Orthop Trauma Surg 2004;124:537–41.
[34] Stannard J, Harris H, McGwin G Jr, et al. Intramedullary nailing of humeral shaft fractures with a locking flexible nail. J Bone Joint Surg Am 2003;85:2103–10.
[35] Heitemeyer U, Kemper F, Hierholzer G, et al. Severely comminuted femoral shaft fractures: treatment by bridging-plate osteosynthesis. Arch Orthop Trauma Surg 1987;106:327–30.
[36] Krettek C, Gerich T, Miclau T. A minimally invasive medial approach for proximal tibial fractures. Injury 2001;32(Suppl 1):SA4–13.
[37] Apivatthakakul T, Arpornchayanon O, Bavornratanavech S. Minimally invasive plate osteosynthesis (MIPO) of the humeral shaft fracture. Is it possible? A cadaveric study and preliminary report. Injury 2005;36:530–8.

ELSEVIER
SAUNDERS

Hand Clin 23 (2007) 449–456

HAND
CLINICS

Humeral Nonunion

Anna R. King, BA, Steven L. Moran, MD, Scott P. Steinmann, MD*

Department of Orthopedic Surgery, Mayo Clinic, 200 First Street SW, Rochester, MN 55902, USA

Humerus fractures comprise 5% to 8% of all fractures [1]. Nonunions are uncommon and can present a frustrating challenge to the orthopedic surgeon. Many methods of treatment have been described with various degrees of success [1]. The rates of healing of humeral nonunions by traditional means of internal fixation with bone graft range from 70% to 92% [2–6], although in cases of infection, poorly vascularized beds, and open, segmental, or severely comminuted fractures, secondary bony healing may still be compromised [7].

Various risk factors may predispose patients to nonunion. Often, patients generally have more than one medical problem, contributing to the poor healing of the fracture. Obesity, osteoporosis, alcoholism, and smoking, among other medical problems, can increase the probability of nonunion, but cannot be corrected before revision surgery [1]. In addition, poor bone quality or bone stock due to arthritis or osteoporosis can further compromise the healing environment. Finally, scar tissue from previous surgical procedures and the proximity of the neurovascular structures to the medial border of the humerus can challenge even experienced surgeons in their attempts at exposing the nonunion site [1,8].

Open reduction and internal fixation (ORIF) combined with autologous bone-grafting can result in reliable healing of the fracture, with a low complication rate [2,9–12]. Not only does the histocompatibility and lack of immunogenicity of an autograft [13,14] complement its osteoinductive and osteoconductive properties [10] but it carries no risk of an autologous graft transmitting occult disease or infection [10,15]. Unfortunately, autograft material does produce some donor site morbidity. In an attempt to avoid this, Hierholzer and colleagues [16] initiated a study to compare the effectiveness of autograft with that of demineralized bone matrix (DBM) in plate fixation of ununited humeral shaft fractures. They found the results regarding fracture healing to be comparable between the two patient groups treated with each of the options. The most effective form of bone graft material, whether autologous, allograft, or synthetic, has yet to be determined through comparative randomized trials.

Not all humeral nonunions are the same. Treatment algorithms are best established by grouping humeral nonunions based on location. Although treatment principles are the same, each fracture location has specific complication rates.

Proximal fractures

Proximal humerus fractures present special problems, and patients generally present with marked disability because of pain and instability [1,17–21]. Most of these fractures are nondisplaced or minimally displaced injuries, which can be managed adequately with closed treatment and early functional rehabilitation [22]. Complications of ORIF of proximal humeral fractures are reported in up to 45% of patients, with avascular necrosis, nonunion, malunion, and nerve injury predominating [23–32]. Acute deep infection after the surgical treatment has also been reported as a rare complication [33].

Several operative techniques have been used to treat these nonunions, including traditional plate-and-screw fixation, blade plates, tension banding, percutaneous pinning, antegrade or retrograde nailing, intramedullary cortical bone grafts, or some combination of these adjunctive procedures

* Corresponding author.
E-mail address: steinmann.scott@mayo.edu (S.P. Steinmann).

doi:10.1016/j.hcl.2007.09.003

[1,34–41]. The osseous architecture of the humeral head, with poor central cancellous bone stock, particularly in elderly patients, has been reported to lead to a high risk of fixation failure with classic plate-and-screw fixation [42–44]. Blade plate fixation, however, may overcome this limitation with the advantage of a fixed-angle device, yet it only affords a single primary proximal point of fixation and can also be technically difficult to insert correctly [1,45]. Both techniques require soft-tissue stripping, with concordant risk to the tenuous vascular supply of the humeral head. Percutaneous pinning and nail fixation allow greater preservation of the soft-tissue envelope and blood supply to the fracture fragments, but the indirect reduction used in these techniques makes anatomic alignment of fracture fragments difficult to achieve [1].

Locking plate fixation appears to provide a good option [46]. It offers the potential advantage of a fixed-angle device with multiple points of proximal fixation, increased load to failure when compared with unlocked plates, increased stability of fixation in osteoporotic bone, and the ability to limit soft-tissue stripping during fracture fixation [1,47].

Scheck [40] used a corticocancellous iliac crest graft in combination with Rush rods on five of his patients, reporting good results overall. Healy and colleagues [35] reported on 25 patients who had proximal humeral nonunions, of whom 14 were initially treated nonoperatively, and 11 treated surgically. The best results of any group were found in those treated with ORIF and bone grafting [1]. Galatz and colleagues [9] recommended ORIF and bone grafting with blade or T-plate fixation, even in older, debilitated patients. Volgas and colleagues [1] treated a small series of proximal humeral nonunions with locking plates, and experienced more failures than successes, explaining that this was probably because these fractures typically place shear across the fracture site, where the locking plate does not add any compression. Ultimately, though, the ideal fixation device for these fractures remains undefined [23], and outcomes can vary on an individual basis.

Diaphyseal fractures

Fractures of the humeral shaft generally heal in 6 to 10 weeks, regardless of treatment. When treated nonoperatively, union rates are reported to be 87% to 100%, and range of motion and pain are minimal. When treated operatively for appropriate indications, the incidence of nonunion is 15% to 30%. Morbidity in the form of shoulder and elbow stiffness, pain, and decreased strength is common [1]. In diaphyseal fractures, the radial nerve frequently may be encased in scar, making it more at risk for iatrogenic injury (Fig. 1) [1].

Open plating, intramedullary nailing, and the use of external fixation have been used in the treatment of these nonunions. With these fractures, insertion of the deltoid limits proximal plating, whereas the olecranon fossa limits distal plating [1]. Of all treatment options, open compression plating and an iliac crest bone graft has been reported to be successful by numerous investigators [1,2,48,49]. The authors found similar results in their practice (Fig. 2). Although autologous cancellous bone grafting is believed to be an important factor contributing to the high union rate achieved with plate-and-screw fixation of ununited diaphyseal fractures [2,11,50–52], it can expose the patient to the discomforts and risks of surgery at the graft donor site [53,54].

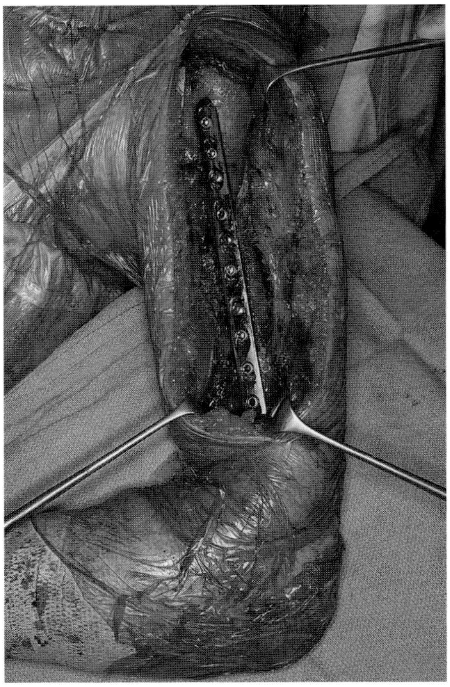

Fig. 1. A 46-year-old man with humerus midshaft nonunion. Treatment with locking plate and iliac crest autograft. The radial nerve required careful dissection from scar at fracture site.

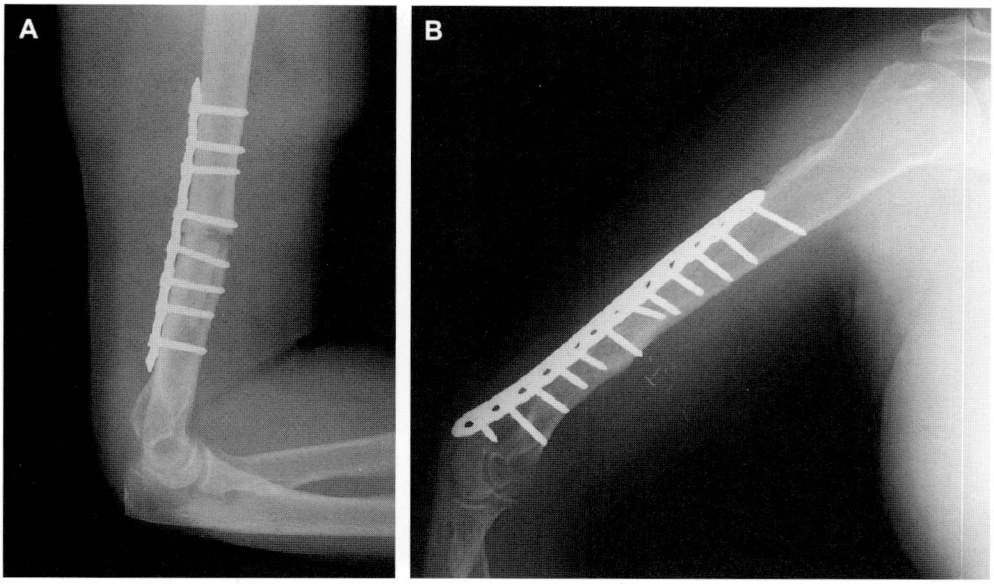

Fig. 2. (*A, B*) A 43-year-old insulin-dependent diabetic with nonunion after posterior plating and iliac crest bone graft. Union achieved after anterolateral plating with locking plate and vascularized medial femoral bone graft.

Distal fractures

Distal humerus fractures can be difficult to bring to union [22,55–67]; often, prior fixation attempts have caused bone loss, which compromises treatment options [1]. Lack of strong cancellous bone, multiple, small distal articular fragments, and complex joint surfaces precluding bicortical fixation can make adequate fixation of these fractures an arduous task [59,61,63,68–70]. These nonunions are often complicated by elbow contracture, articular deterioration, poor bone stock, retained hardware, and ulnar nerve problems [1,58,71,72].

Many treatment options have been described, including ORIF with plates and screws [11,51,73–75], intramedullary nailing with interfragmentary wiring [76], elbow arthroplasty [77], free vascularized bone grafting [5], neurolysis, contracture release, or a combination of these procedures [11,57,75,76,78]. Compression plating is preferred in most circumstances.

ORIF is typically recommended for treatment of uninfected nonunions in younger, more active patients who have good bone stock at the injury site [55,72,77]. In a subset of patients, the bone may be too osteoporotic for traditional fixation techniques [8]. The rate of bony union following ORIF in the treatment of uninfected distal humeral nonunions has been reported to range from 64% to 100% [11,57,58,77–80], but the presence of infection is often associated with lower rates of successful bony union, limited fixation options, and worse functional outcomes [1,4,58]. Treatment of infected nonunions, particularly those that have failed in multiple attempts at internal fixation or that have significant deformity, is complex (Fig. 3) [72,81].

Special considerations in the elderly

Geriatric patients who have osteopenic bone generally require different strategies from the traditional treatment philosophies and techniques. Most physicians agree that elderly patients are served best by rapid, definitive fracture care, aimed at early restoration of function, and achieved by anatomic restoration of the articular surface, stable fixation, and early motion [8]. Fracture union, rather than motion, is the first priority in these cases, because motion can be restored reliably by subsequent contracture release, if necessary, as long as the fracture heals [8]. In this sense, inadequate internal fixation combined with early mobilization may lead to nonunion and loss of bone stock [11,82–84].

Bone grafting

The choice of bone graft material still remains controversial. Although iliac crest has remained the gold standard, newer options for grafting may achieve better or equivalent results, with less donor site morbidity. The recent study by Hierholzer and

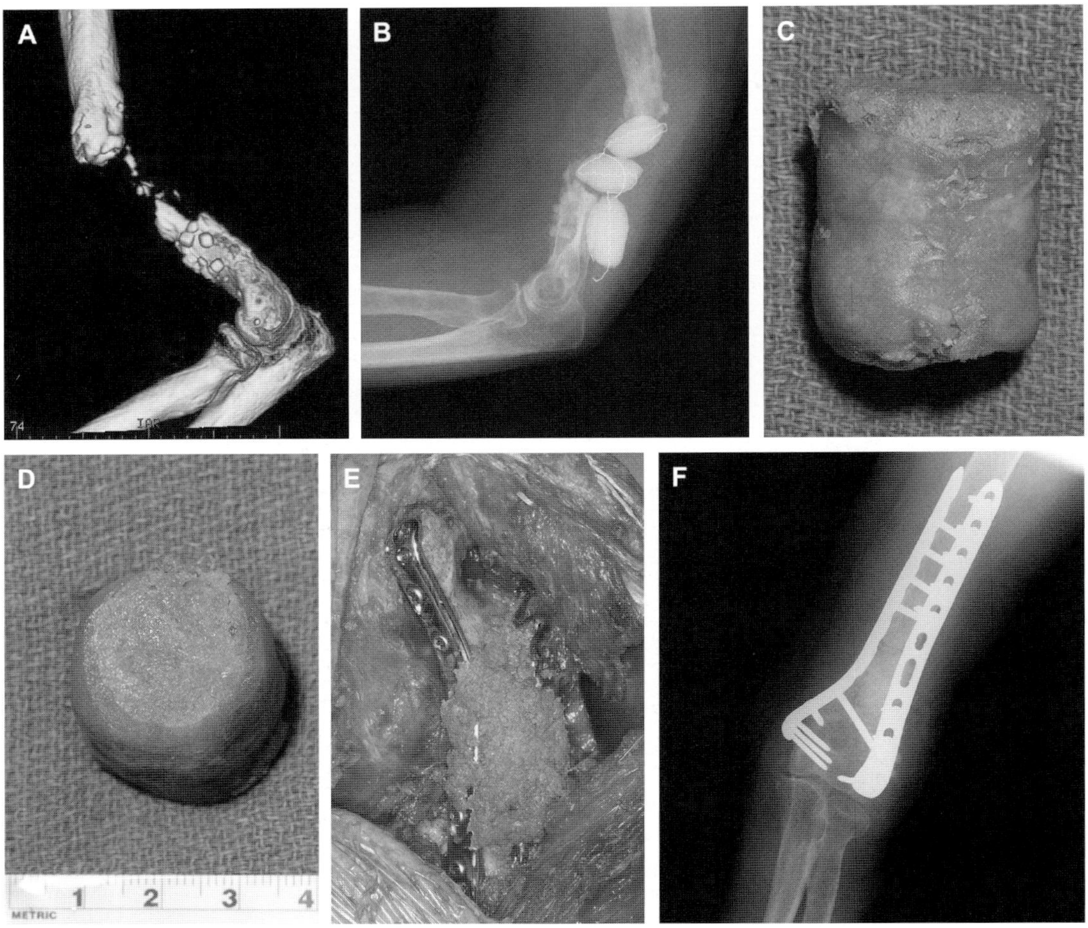

Fig. 3. (*A* and *B*) A 50-year-old woman who was a smoker, with chronic infected nonunion after two prior attempts at fixation. (*C*, *D*, and *E*) Bone graft obtained from the femoral canal and wrapped with an Infuse graft was placed into the defect after debridement with antibiotic spacer. (*F*) Patient at 2 months postoperative, demonstrating healed fracture.

colleagues [16] looked at the effect of bone graft on the healing of ununited humeral shaft fractures. They compared DBM to autografts and found that DBM proved to be effective for augmenting the surgical repair; the healing and clinical outcome was comparable with that following augmentation with autograft. They argued that DBM, in particular, can be used for standard graft augmentation, in an effort to avoid the harvest of an iliac bone graft and its associated donor-site morbidity [16]. Use of autologous bone graft requires an additional surgical site and increased surgical time, and it is often associated with multiple complications [53,85–87] that are not seen with the use of DBM.

Vascularized periosteal bone flaps from the iliac crest, distal humerus, tenth rib, and distal femur have been used previously in the treatment of bony nonunions, avascular necrosis, osteoradionecrosis, osteomyelitis, and reconstruction of bone defects (Fig. 4) [7,88–91]. Recently, femoral condylar grafts used for the treatment of recalcitrant nonunions within the extremities have been described. Although some have shown the periosteum to be osteogenic, others have found that periosteal grafts are unreliable when harvested without their cortical components [7,92–95] because the fine cambium layer of the isolated graft is easily injured when the periosteum is separated from the cortex, thus suppressing the osteogenic effects of the flap [7,96]. However, when a small piece of cortical bone is included in the graft, the "corticoperiosteal" graft maintains its bone-forming ability [97]. As opposed to a vascularized fibular graft, the medial femoral condylar periosteal flap is smaller, more flexible, and may be easily tailored to irregular

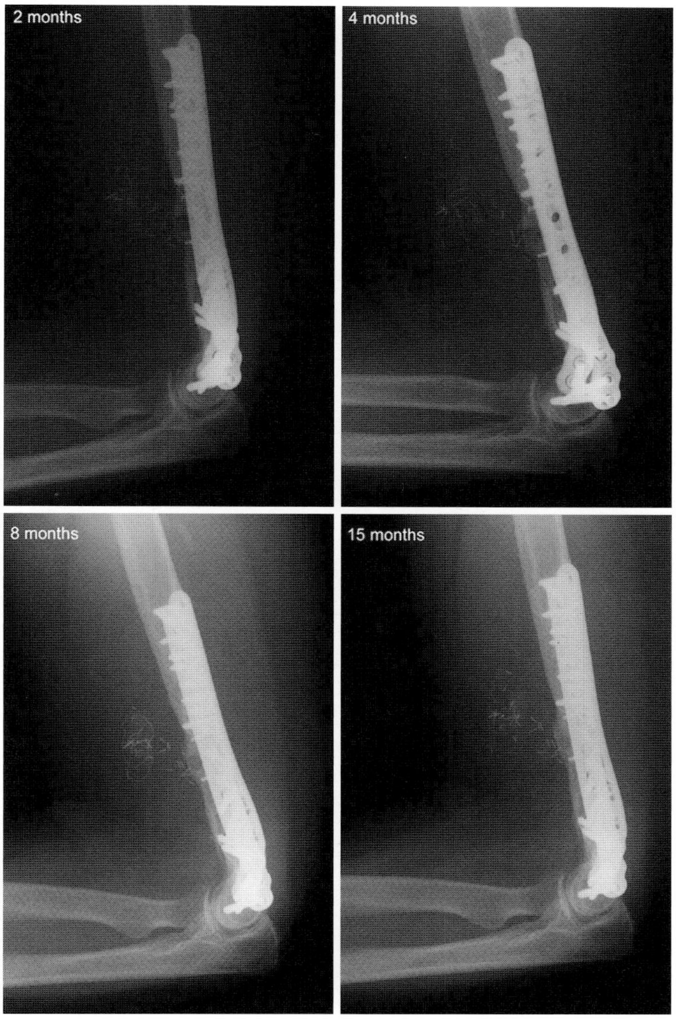

Fig. 4. Patient with nonunion of humeral shaft salvaged with vascularized medial femoral bone graft. Sequential radiographs show union over 15 months.

defects. The elasticity of the flap allows for a tighter fit around a tubular bone; it is especially useful in areas of small defect, where the use of a fibular or iliac crest flap may be unwarranted. The authors have treated five patients successfully with a vascularized corticoperiosteal bone flap from the medial femoral supracondylar region for humeral nonunion. The average time to union was 7.5 months, and none of the cases required subsequent revisions. All four patients had excellent shoulder and elbow function.

References

[1] Volgas D, Stannard J, Alonso J. Nonunions of the humerus. Clin Orthop Relat Res 2004;419:46–50.

[2] Healy WL, White GL, Mick CA, et al. Nonunion of the humeral shaft. Clin Orthop 1987;219: 206–13.

[3] Ebraheim NA, Mekhail AO, Darwich M. Open reduction and internal fixation with bone grafting of clavicular nonunion. J Trauma 1997;42: 701–4.

[4] Haidukewych GJ, Sperling JW. Results of treatment of infected humeral nonunions: the mayo clinic experience. Clin Orthop 2003;414:25–30.

[5] Beredjiklian PK, Hotchkiss RN, Athanasian EA, et al. Recalcitrant nonunion of the distal humerus: treatment with free vascularized bone grafting. Clin Orthop 2005;435:134–9.

[6] Wood MB. Free vascularized bone transfers for nonunions, segmental gaps, and following tumor resection. Orthopedics 1986;9:810–6.

[7] Doi K, Sakai K. Vascularized periosteal bone graft from the supracondylar region of the femur. Microsurgery 1994;15(5):305–15.
[8] Hausman M, Panozzo A. Treatment of distal humerus fractures in the elderly. Clin Orthop Relat Res 2004;425:55–63.
[9] Galatz L, Williams GR Jr, Fenlin JM Jr, et al. Outcome of open reduction and internal fixation of surgical neck nonunions of the humerus. J Orthop Trauma 2004;18(2):63–7.
[10] Friedlaender G. Bone grafts. The basic science rationale for clinical applications. J Bone Joint Surg Am 1987;69:786–90.
[11] Helfet D, Kloen P, Anand N, et al. Open reduction and internal fixation of delayed unions and nonunions of fractures of the distal part of the humerus. J Bone Joint Surg Am 2003;85:33–40.
[12] Helfet D, Jupiter J, Gasser S. Indirect reduction and tension-band plating of tibial nonunion with deformity. J Bone Joint Surg Am 1992;74:1286–97.
[13] Bolano L, Kopta J. The immunology of bone and cartilage transplantation. Orthopedics 1991;14: 987–96.
[14] Horowitz M, Friedlaender G. Immunologic aspects of bone transplantation. A rationale for future studies. Orthop Clin North Am 1987;18:227–33.
[15] Chapman P, Villar R. The bacteriology of bone allografts. J Bone Joint Surg Am 1992;74:398–9.
[16] Hierholzer C, Sama D, Toro JB, et al. Plate fixation of ununited humeral shaft fractures: effect of type of bone graft on healing. J Bone Joint Surg 2006;88:1442–7.
[17] Antuna S, Sperling JW, Sanchez-Sotelo J, et al. Shoulder arthroplasty for proximal humeral malunions: long-term results. J Shoulder Elbow Surg 2002;11(2):122–9.
[18] Naranja RJ, Lannotti J. Displaced three- and four-part proximal humerus fractures: evaluation and management. J Am Acad Orthop Surg 2000;8: 373–82.
[19] Wijgman A, Roolker W, Patt TW, et al. Open reduction and internal fixation of three and four-part fractures of the proximal part of the humerus. J Bone Joint Surg Am 2002;84:1919–25.
[20] Court-Brown C, Cattermole H, McQueen M. Impacted valgus fractures (B1.1) of the proximal humerus: the results of non-operative treatment. J Bone Joint Surg Am 2002;84:504–8.
[21] Court-Brown C, Garg A, McQueen M. The translated two-part fracture of the proximal humerus: epidemiology and outcome in the older patient. J Bone Joint Surg Am 2001;83:799–804.
[22] Kaplan F. Form and function of bone. In: Simone SR, editor. Orthopaedic basic science. Rosemont (IL): American Academy of Orthopaedic Surgeons; 1994. p. 127–84.
[23] Connor P, Flatow E. Complications of internal fixation of proximal humeral fractures. Instr Course Lect 1997;46:25–37.
[24] de Laat E, Visser CP, Coene LN, et al. Nerve lesions in primary shoulder dislocations and humeral neck fractures. A prospective clinical and EMG study. J Bone Joint Surg Am 1994;76:381–3.
[25] Flatow E. Fractures of the proximal humerus. In: Bucholz RW, Heckman JD, editors. Rockwood and Green's fractures in adults. 5th edition. Philadelphia: Lippincott, WIlliams and Wilkins; 2001. p. 1028–40.
[26] Gerber C, Werner C, Vienne P. Internal fixation of complex fractures of the proximal humerus. J Bone Joint Surg Am 2004;86:848–55.
[27] Misra A, Kapur R, Maffulli N. Complex proximal humeral fractures in adults: a systematic review of management. Injury 2001;32:363–72.
[28] Moda S, Chadha NS, Sangwan SS, et al. Open reduction and fixation of proximal humeral fractures and fracture-dislocations. J Bone Joint Surg Am 1990;72:1050–2.
[29] Neer C II. Displaced proximal humeral fractures II. Treatment of three-part and four-part displacement. J Bone Joint Surg Am 1970;52:1090–103.
[30] Szyszkowitz R, Seggl W, Schleifer P, et al. Proximal humeral fractures. Management techniques and expected results. Clin Orthop Relat Res 1993;(292): 13–25.
[31] Wirth M. Late sequelae of proximal humerus fractures. Instr Course Lect 2003;52:13–6.
[32] Zyto K, Ahrengart L, Sperber A, et al. Treatment of displaced proximal humeral fractures in elderly patients. J Bone Joint Surg Am 1997;79:412–7.
[33] Athwal G, Sperling JW, Rispoli DM, et al. Acute deep infection after surgical fixation or proximal humeral fractures. J Shoulder Elbow Surg 2007;16(4):408–12.
[34] Duralde X, Flatow EL, Pollock RG, et al. Operative treatment of nonunions of the surgical neck of the humerus. J Shoulder Elbow Surg 1996;5:169–80.
[35] Healy W, Jupiter JB, Kristiansen TK, et al. Nonunions of the proximal humerus: a review of 25 cases. J Orthop Trauma 1990;4:424–31.
[36] Jupiter J, Mullaji A. Blade plate fixation of proximal humeral non-unions. Injury 1994;25:301–3.
[37] Kristiansen B, Christensen S. Proximal humeral fractures. Acta Orthop Scand 1987;58:124–7.
[38] Nayak N, Schickendantz MS, Regan WD, et al. Operative treatment of nonunion of surgical neck fractures of the humerus. Clin Orthop 1995;313:200–5.
[39] Ring D, McKee MD, Perey BH, et al. The use of a blade plate and autogenous cancellous bone graft in the treatment of ununited fractures of the proximal humerus. J Shoulder Elbow Surg 2001;10:501–7.
[40] Scheck M. Surgical treatment of nonunions of the surgical neck of the humerus. Clin Orthop 1982; 167:255–9.
[41] Walch G, Badet R, Nove-Josserand L, et al. Nonunions of the surgical neck of the humerus: surgical treatment with an intramedullary bone peg, internal fixation, and cancellous bone grafting. J Shoulder Elbow Surg 1996;5:161–8.

[42] Hall M, Rosser M. The structure of the upper end of the humerus with reference to osteoporotic changes in senescence leading to fractures. Can Med Assoc J 1963;88:290–4.

[43] Hawkins R, Bell R, Gurr K. The three-part fracture of the proximal part of the humerus, operative treatment. J Bone Joint Surg Am 1986;68:1410–4.

[44] Kristiansen T, Christensen S. Plate fixation of proximal humeral fractures. Acta Orthop Scand 1986;57:320–3.

[45] Instrum K, Fennell C, Shrive N, et al. Semitubular blade plate fixation in proximal humeral fractures: a biomechanical study in a cadaveric model. J Shoulder Elbow Surg 1998;7:462–6.

[46] Rose P, Adams CR, Torchia ME, et al. Locking plate fixation for proximal humeral fractures: initial results with a new implant. J Shoulder Elbow Surg 2007;16(2):202–7.

[47] Haidukewych G. Perspectives on modern orthopaedics: innovations in locking plate technology. J Am Acad Orthop Surg 2004;12:205–12.

[48] Barquet A, Fernandez A, Luvizio J, et al. A combined therapeutic protocol for aseptic nonunion of the humeral shaft: a report of 25 cases. J Trauma 1989;29:95–8.

[49] Rodriguez-Merchan C, Gomez-Castresana F. Internal fixation of nonunions. Clin Orthop Relat Res 2004;419:13–20.

[50] Marti R, Verheyen C, Besselaar P. Humeral shaft nonunion: evaluation of uniform surgical repair in 51 patients. J Orthop Trauma 2002;16:108–15.

[51] Helfet D, Kloen P, Anand N, et al. ORIF of delayed unions and nonunions of distal humeral fractures. Surgical technique. J Bone Joint Surg Am 2004; 86(Suppl 1):18–29.

[52] Ring D, Jupiter JB, Quintero J, et al. Atrophic ununited diaphyseal fractures of the humerus with a bony defect: treatment by wave-plate osteosynthesis. J Bone Joint Surg Br 2000;82:867–71.

[53] Arrington E, Smith WJ, Chambers HG, et al. Complications of iliac crest graft harvesting. Clin Orthop Relat Res 1996;329:300–9.

[54] Goulet J, Senunas LE, DeSilva GL, et al. Autogenous iliac crest bone graft. Complications and functional assessment. Clin Orthop Relat Res 1997;339:76–81.

[55] Ackerman G, Jupiter J. Non-union of fractures of the distal end of the humerus. J Bone Joint Surg Am 1988;70:75–83.

[56] Masada K, Kawai H, Kawabata H, et al. Osteosynthesis for old, established non-union of the lateral condyle of the humerus. J Bone Joint Surg Am 1990;72:32–40.

[57] Sanders R, Sackett J. Open reduction and internal fixation of delayed union and nonunion of the distal humerus. J Orthop Trauma 1990;4:254–9.

[58] Brinker M, O'Connor DP, Crouch CC, et al. Ilizarov treatment of infected nonunions of the distal humerus after failure of internal fixation: an outcomes study. J Orthop Trauma 2007;21(3):178–84.

[59] Gabel G, Hanson G, Bennett JB, et al. Intraarticular fractures of the distal humerus in the adult. Clin Orthop 1987;219:99–108.

[60] Henley M, Bone L, Parker B. Operative management of intra-articular fractures of the distal humerus. J Orthop Trauma 1987;1:24–35.

[61] Holdsworth B, Mossad M. Fractures of the adult distal humerus: elbow function after internal fixation. J Bone Joint Surg Br 1990;72:362–5.

[62] John H, Rosso R, Neff U, et al. Operative treatment of distal humeral fractures in the elderly. J Bone Joint Surg Br 1994;76:793–6.

[63] Letsch R, Schmit-Neuerburg KP, Sturmer KM, et al. Intraarticular fractures of the distal humerus: surgical treatment and results. Clin Orthop 1984;241:238–44.

[64] O'Driscoll S, S-SJ, Torchia M. Management of the smashed distal humerus. Orthop Clin North Am 2002;33:19–33.

[65] Helfet D, Hotchkiss RN. Internal fixation of the distal humerus: a biomechanical comparison of methods. J Orthop Trauma 1990;4:260–4.

[66] Ring D, Jupiter J. Fractures of the distal humerus. Orthop Clin North Am 2000;31:103–13.

[67] Self J, Viegas SF, Buford WL Jr, et al. A comparison of double-plate fixation methods for complex distal humerus fractures. J Shoulder Elbow Surg 1995;4: 10–6.

[68] Caja V, Moroni A, Vendemia V, et al. Surgical treatment of bicondylar fractures of the distal humerus. Injury 1994;25:433–8.

[69] Jupiter J, Neff U, Holzach P, et al. Intercondylar fractures of the humerus. J Bone Joint Surg Am 1985;67:226–39.

[70] Wang K, Shih HN, Hsu KY, et al. Intercondylar fractures of the distal humerus: routine anterior subcutaneous transposition of the ulnar nerve in a posterior operative approach. J Trauma 1994;36:770–3.

[71] Ring D, Jupiter J, Toh S. Salvage of contaminated fractures of the distal humerus with thin wire external fixation. Clin Orthop Relat Res 1999;359:203–8.

[72] Pugh D, McKee M. Advances in the management of humeral nonunion. J Am Acad Orthop Surg 2003; 11:48–59.

[73] Jupiter J. Complex fractures of the distal part of the humerus and associated complications. Instr Course Lect 1995;44:187–98.

[74] Harvey E, Henley MB, Swiontkowski MF, et al. The use of a locking custom contoured blade plate for peri-articular nonunions. Injury 2003;34:111–6.

[75] Ring D, Gulotta L, Jupiter J. Unstable nonunions of the distal part of the humerus. J Bone Joint Surg Am 2003;85:1040–6.

[76] Lin J, Chiang H, Chang D. Locked nailing with interfragmentary wiring for humeral nonunions. J Trauma 2002;52:733–8.

[77] Morrey B, Adams R. Semiconstrained elbow replacement for distal humeral nonunion. J Bone Joint Surg Am 1995;7:67–72.

[78] McKee M, Jupiter J, Toh CL, et al. Reconstruction after malunion and nonunion of intra-articular fractures of the distal humerus. Methods and results in 13 adults. J Bone Joint Surg Am 1994;76:614–21.
[79] Ali A, Douglas H, Stanley D. Revision surgery for nonunion after early failure of fixation of fractures of the distal humerus. J Bone Joint Surg Am 2005;87: 1107–10.
[80] Mitsunaga M, Bryan R, Linscheid R. Condylar nonunions of the elbow. J Trauma 1982;22:787–91.
[81] Pugh D, Rozbruch S. Nonunions and malunions. In: Baumgaertner MR, Tornetta P, editors. Orthopaedic knowledge update trauma 3. Rosemont (IL): American Academy of Orthopaedic Surgeons; 2005. p. 115–30.
[82] Morrey B. Fractures of the distal humerus: role of elbow replacement. Orthop Clin North Am 2000;31:145–54.
[83] Morrey B. Post-traumatic contracture of the elbow. J Bone Joint Surg Am 1990;72:601–18.
[84] Nowicki K, Shall L. Arthroscopic release of a post-traumatic flexion contracture of the elbow: a case report and review of the literature. Arthroscopy 1992;8:544–7.
[85] Wilkins R, Kelly C. The effect of allomatrix injectable putty on the outcome of long bone applications. Orthopedics 2003;26(Suppl 5):s567–70.
[86] Sommer C, Gautier E, Muller M, et al. First clinical results of the locking compression plate (LCP). Injury 2003;34(Suppl 2):B43–54.
[87] Constant C, Murley A. A clinical method of functional assessment of the shoulder. Clin Orthop Relat Res 1987;214:160–4.
[88] King KF. Periosteal pedicle grafting in dogs. J Bone Joint Surg Br 1976;58:117–21.
[89] Fuchs B, Steinmann P, Bishop AT. Free vascularized corticoperiosteal bone graft for the treatment of persistent nonunion of the clavicle. J Shoulder Elbow Surg 2005;14:264–8.
[90] Kobayashi S, Kakibuchi M, Masuda T, et al. Use of vascularized corticoperiosteal flap from the femur for reconstruction of the orbit. Ann Plast Surg 1994;33(4):351–7 [discussion: 357–58].
[91] Stock W, Hierner R, Wolf K. [Vascularized periosteal transplant. A review of a new therapeutic possibility]. Handchir Mikrochir Plast Chir 1991;23(3): 149–56 [in German].
[92] Skoog T. The use of periosteal flaps in the repair of clefts of the primary palate. Cleft Palate J 1965;2: 332–9.
[93] Takato T, Harii K, Nakatsuka T, et al. Vascularized periosteal grafts: an experimental study using two different forms of tibial periosteum in rabbits. Plast Reconstr Surg 1986;78(4):489–97.
[94] Finley JM, Acland RD, Wood MB. Revascularized periosteal grafts–a new method to produce functional new bone without bone grafting. Plast Reconstr Surg 1978;61(1):1–6.
[95] Acland RD. Caution about clinical use of vascularized periosteal grafts. Plast Reconstr Surg 1978; 62(2):290.
[96] Sakai K, Doi K, Kawai S. Free vascularized thin corticoperiosteal graft. Plast Reconstr Surg 1991; 87(2):290–8.
[97] Del Pinal F, et al. Vascularized corticoperiosteal grafts from the medial femoral condyle for difficult non-unions of the upper limb. J Hand Surg [Br] 2007;32E(2):135–42 [European volume].

ELSEVIER
SAUNDERS

Hand Clin 23 (2007) 457–469

HAND
CLINICS

Distal Humerus Fractures

Thomas W. Throckmorton, MD, Peter C. Zarkadas, MD,
Scott P. Steinmann, MD*

Mayo Clinic, Department of Orthopedic Surgery, 200 First Street SW, Rochester, MN 55902, USA

Fractures of the distal humerus in adults have traditionally presented a treatment challenge for the orthopedic surgeon. The combination of anatomic complexity, multifragmentary comminution, and a short distal segment, often in the setting of osteoporotic bone, renders these fractures difficult to treat successfully and often make a full restoration of function uncertain. Multiple methods of treatment for these fractures have been described, including bracing, internal fixation, hemiarthroplasty, and total elbow arthroplasty (TEA).

This article reviews the epidemiology and classification of these injuries and the numerous described fixation and arthroplasty techniques. The current treatment algorithm and authors' preferred method of internal fixation are also illustrated. Additionally, the treatment of these injuries in the elderly population and the complications of surgical treatment are reviewed.

Epidemiology

Population-based studies have established our baseline understanding of distal humerus fractures. Robinson and colleagues [1] reported a 5.7/100,000 prevalence of these injuries, with a bimodal distribution regarding gender and age. The first peak occurred in boys/men aged 12 to 19, followed by a second peak in women older than 80. The prevalence in men decreased in the third through sixth decades before increasing again after age 70. The prevalence in women increased every decade after age 20. Older patients were typically injured in falls, whereas younger individuals sustained their fractures more commonly during athletic activities or motor vehicle accidents (Fig. 1).

A similar study conducted at the authors' institution from 1965 to 1974 described the incidence of all humerus fractures seen over a 10-year period. Of 586 humerus fractures, 191 (33%) involved the distal third. These fractures were most commonly seen in a younger population. However, incidence also increased with age. Between ages 50 and 69, 11 fractures per 100,000 person-years were reported, which increased to 21 fractures per 100,000 person-years in the group aged 70 and older. The mechanism of injury was typically a fall from height or significant trauma [2].

With regard to the elderly population, the prevalence of these injuries continues to rise. A study of osteoporotic distal humerus fractures in elderly women over a 25-year period documented an increasing prevalence, from 11/100,000 in 1970 to 30/100,000 in 1995. The age-adjusted prevalence increased similarly over the same time period. A regression analysis based on these data predicted a prevalence of 52/100,000 women by the year 2030, which would reflect an exponential growth of these injuries [3]. The investigators called for preventive measures to stem this growing trend.

Clinical evaluation

As with all injuries, the evaluation begins with a thorough history and physical examination. Careful attention must be paid to the mechanism of injury, which denotes the amount of energy absorbed by the affected limb. The physical

* Corresponding author.
E-mail address: Steinmann.Scott@mayo.edu (S.P. Steinmann).

doi:10.1016/j.hcl.2007.09.001

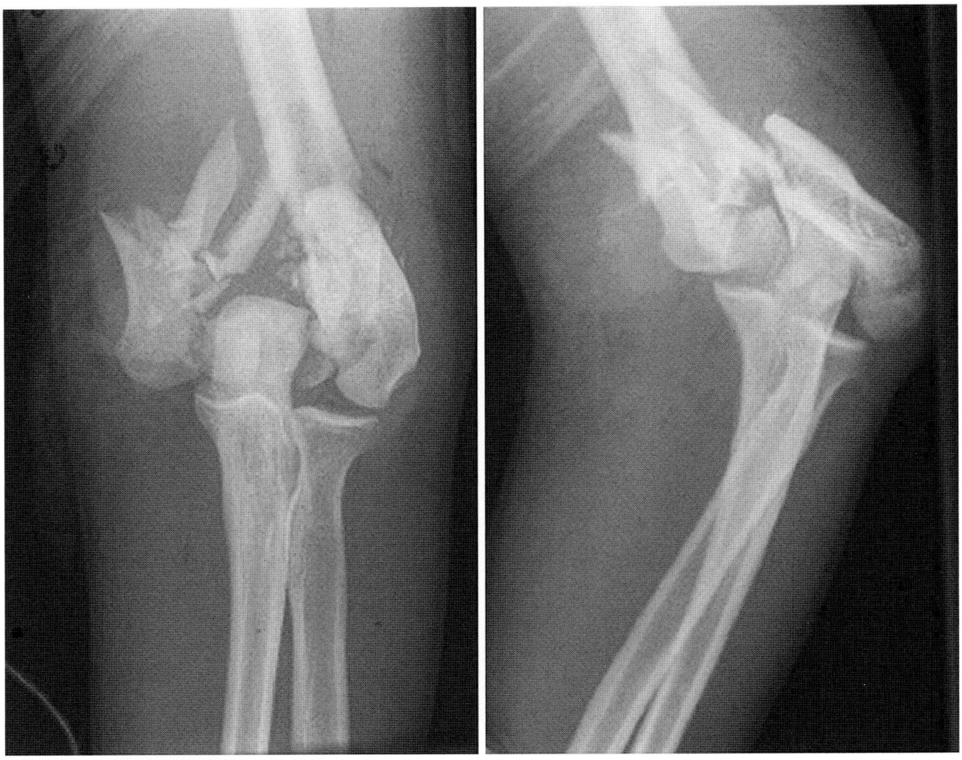

Fig. 1. Distal humerus fractures often are the result of significant trauma in young adult patients. In the elderly, however, they are more commonly seen after a lower energy mechanism, such as a fall.

examination should include assessment of the skin and soft tissues to reveal the presence of an open injury or significant soft tissue damage. Although neurovascular disruption is thought to be uncommon with these fractures, a complete evaluation of these structures should be performed to rule out any such injuries.

Classification

The most commonly referenced classification system for adult distal humerus fractures was advanced by Muller (Fig. 2) [4]. Known as the Orthopedic Trauma Association classification, this scheme categorizes these fractures anatomically. Type A injuries include extra-articular, transcondylar, and apophyseal fractures. Type B fractures have partial articular involvement, whereas type C injuries have complete or complex involvement of the elbow joint.

Other classification systems have also been described. The system of Mehne and Matta was advanced in 1992. In this scheme, type I fractures are intra-articular and are subdivided into single- and double-column fractures. Capitellar and trochlear fractures are also treated separately under this category. Type II fractures are extra-articular but intracapsular. These fractures include high (proximal to the olecranon fossa) and low (involving the olecranon fossa) transcondylar fractures. Type III fractures are extracapsular and essentially are those that involve the medial or lateral epicondyles [5].

In another submitted classification scheme, Davies and Stanley achieved substantial intraobserver and interobserver agreement with their radiographically based system that defines fractures as extra-articular, predominantly intra-articular, or predominantly articular [6].

Adding CT has also been found to be helpful in fracture classification. A recent study by Doornberg and colleagues [7] found that reformatting images with three-dimensional CT substantially improved intraobserver reliability but did not significantly affect interobserver agreement. The investigators also concluded that this addition was a helpful adjunct for preoperative planning.

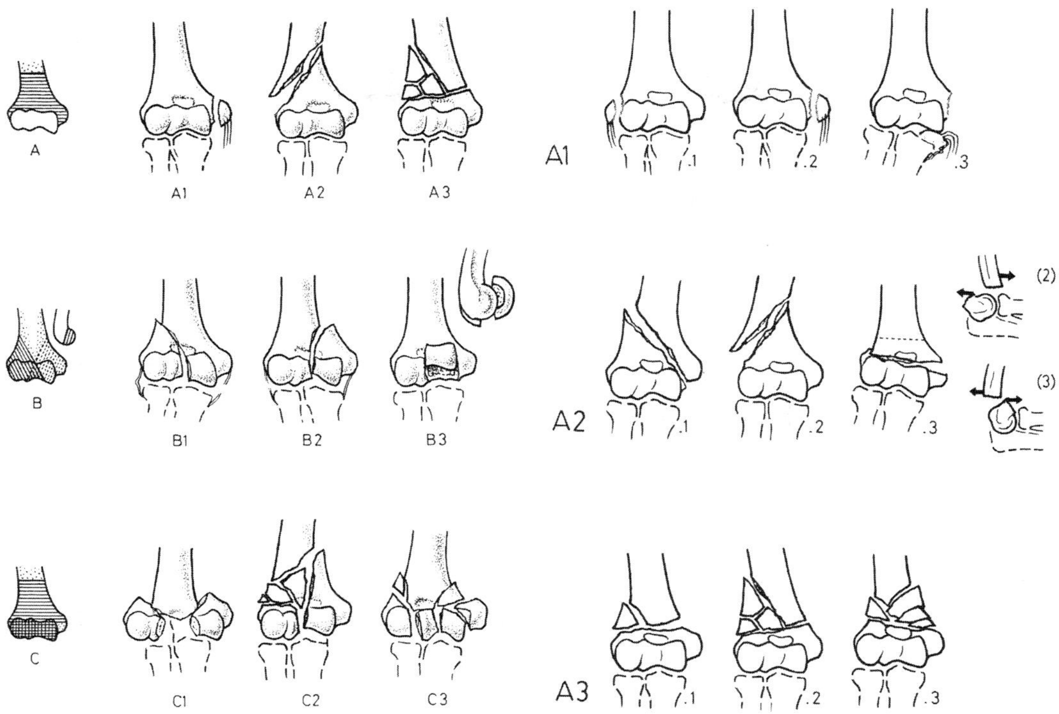

Fig. 2. AO classification of distal humerus fractures (*Adapted from* Muller ME, Koch P, Schaftzker J. Comprehensive classification of fractures of long bones. Berlin: Springer-Verlag; 1990; with permission.)

Conservative treatment

Although much of the current literature has focused on the operative treatment of these fractures, some investigators have advocated conservative treatment for extra-articular injuries. Sarmiento and colleagues [8] published a series of 85 such fractures treated with bracing. Although 15% of the fractures were open and 18% had peripheral nerve injuries at presentation, functional bracing resulted in 96% union, no infections, and good functional results. All nerve injuries also had resolved or were improving at the time of latest follow-up.

Another recent study showed similarly good outcomes after functional bracing of distal third humeral shaft fractures (ie, extra-articular) in young adults. In this series, all 21 fractures united, with minimal angular deformity and no restriction in elbow motion [9].

Operative versus nonoperative treatment

Early studies comparing operative and nonoperative treatment for adult distal humerus fractures often concluded that conservative treatment was superior. Horne [10] reported in a series of 50 patients that better results were obtained with nonoperative than with operative treatment. The poor results of surgical treatment were attributed to an inability to maintain rigid fixation, which resulted in a lengthy period of immobilization. Conservative treatment was recommended for all but the simplest distal humerus fractures.

Other studies of the same period, although acknowledging the technical challenge of obtaining secure distal fixation, tended to favor operative fixation when possible. In one report of 24 comminuted distal humerus fractures, better functional results were obtained with surgical intervention than with nonoperative treatment. Conservative therapy was recommended in cases where adequate fixation could not be attained or in contaminated wounds [11]. Further, Zagorski and others [12] compared operative and nonoperative treatment in 42 comminuted intra-articular distal humerus fractures. Patients treated with open reduction internal fixation achieved 76% good and excellent results, whereas only 8% of patients obtained the same outcome with conservative treatment. These investigators concluded that rigid anatomic fixation combined with early motion were associated with favorable results. These fundamental principles continue to govern our currently accepted treatment paradigm for these injuries. As such, internal fixation is generally accepted as the standard of care for the treatment of intra-articular distal humerus fractures.

Operative fixation

Initial failures of internal fixation for adult distal humerus fractures were typically related to an inability to achieve rigid fixation, particularly in the distal segment, which is often comminuted or osteoporotic. However, Gabel and colleagues [13] in 1987 published a report of 13 patients who had distal humerus fractures treated with dual plating. Of the 10 patients available at 2 years of follow-up, 9 of them attained good or excellent results. Based on these data, the investigators advocated operative treatment with their technique to allow rigid fixation and early motion.

In the early 1990s, Helfet and Schmeling [14] advanced a protocol consisting of orthogonal medial column and posterior lateral column plating for intra-articular distal humerus fractures. With this technique, they attained 75% good and excellent results for Muller type C fractures, and a low complication rate. On the basis of these results, fixation of adult distal humerus fractures for the past 15 years has focused on this concept of "90-90" plating.

More recently, multiple fixation techniques have been described. These include fixation using custom T-plates [15], double tension-band plating [16], lateral J-plates [17], minifragment osteosynthesis [18], Kirschner wires [19], large fragment tibial plates [20], and reconstruction plates [21]. All these fixation methods have achieved some manner of success using objective or subjective outcome measures. Additionally, augmentation using tricortical iliac crest bone graft has been advocated for particularly comminuted fractures [22].

Biomechanics of fixation

With the realization that rigid fixation is difficult to attain in the distal humerus, several investigators have analyzed the biomechanical features of different plate configurations. Self and colleagues [23] reported their results with medial and lateral plating using supplementation with bolts. They found this configuration to have increased strength and stability compared with other constructs.

Subsequently, Jacobsen and colleagues [24] reported their biomechanical data in testing different plate configurations. They found no difference in torsional stiffness among the different constructs tested. All constructs were susceptible to bending stress in the sagittal plane, compared with intact specimens. The configuration of a medial pelvic reconstruction plate combined with a posterolateral dynamic compression plate achieved the strongest sagittal plane stiffness. Adding a third plate laterally did not add any significant resistance to bending.

With the advent of locking plate technology, attention turned toward testing the biomechanical properties of these devices in distal humerus fractures. One study concluded that locking compression plates confer "substantial advantage" in these fractures when the bone quality is poor or if significant metaphyseal comminution is present [25]. The same investigator later reported the results of a cadaveric study testing locking compression plates versus reconstruction plates in orthogonal and parallel posterior configurations. In this model, an increase in stiffness to torsional and anteroposterior bending forces was reported with a construct using locking plates at a 90° orientation to each other. However, plate types showed little difference in stiffness, and the investigators concluded that plate configuration was a more important variable than plate type. Nevertheless, they also suggested that locking plates may be helpful in the setting of osteoporosis or comminution [26].

Operative approaches

One area of controversy in these fractures is the use of the olecranon osteotomy to attain full exposure of the distal humerus and elbow joint. Advocates point to the relative ease of fixation without the triceps obstructing the surgeon's view, whereas detractors are often concerned with the small, but not insignificant, rate of osteotomy nonunion. Coles and colleagues [27] described their 6-year experience with distal humerus fractures using olecranon osteotomy, particularly for more complex fractures. They encountered no nonunions in their series of 67 patients, despite the fact that more than one half of these fractures were open. Five patients (8%) required isolated hardware removal for symptomatic discomfort. The investigators recommended the use of olecranon osteotomy for complex intra-articular distal humerus fractures. Another study advocates preservation of the anconeus by lifting it as a flap before olecranon osteotomy (Fig. 3) [28]. Standard olecranon osteotomy approaches result in denervation of the anconeus muscle, which should be avoided.

As an alternative, the entire triceps and anconeus can be reflected as a unit off the olecranon [29,30]. Although this approach provides adequate exposure for all types of distal humerus fractures, concern exists about the ultimate healing of the triceps back to the olecranon bony surface.

Other investigators have used a triceps-splitting exposure in these fractures, which can be a difficult exposure for type C fractures for most orthopedic surgeons, but has been shown to be useful in at least one report [31]. In a series of 33 distal humerus fractures (29 of which were type C) with a mean of 26 months follow-up, Ziran and colleagues [31] concluded that a triceps-splitting approach allowed adequate exposure, with an acceptable rate of complications.

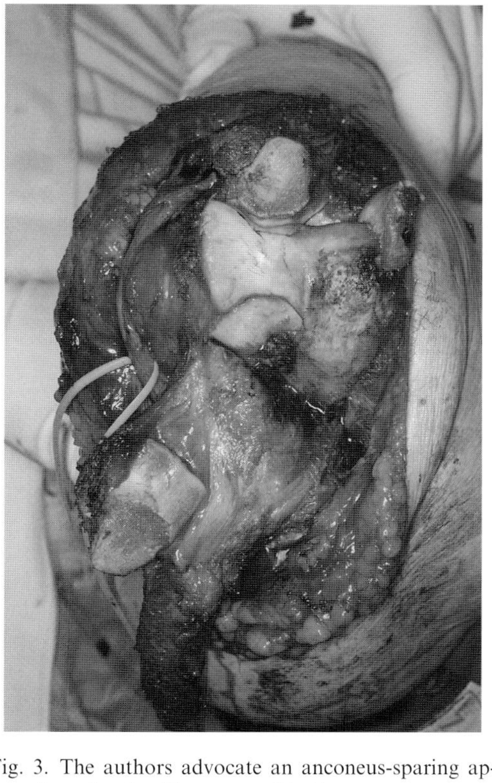

Fig. 3. The authors advocate an anconeus-sparing approach to the distal humerus with olecranon osteotomy for exposure of intra-articular distal humerus fractures.

Ulnar nerve management

Ulnar neuropathy is a well-recognized postoperative complication of adult distal humerus fractures, and routine transposition of the nerve is routinely advocated [32,33]. Wang and colleagues [33] reported the results of 20 patients who had distal humerus fractures treated with open reduction internal fixation and anterior subcutaneous ulnar nerve transposition. In a follow-up period ranging from 15 to 35 months, no patients had ulnar nerve symptoms. The investigators recommended routine transposition to avoid postoperative ulnar neuritis.

Other investigators have not routinely transposed the ulnar nerve and have reported their results. Gupta [34] reported on a series of 55 distal humerus fractures treated with posterior fixation. Only one patient underwent coincident ulnar nerve transposition. Three patients developed ulnar neuritis, which resolved by the third postoperative week. Although this report indicates that ulnar nerve transposition is not mandatory with dual posterior plating constructs, the authors would argue that constructs involving the use of a medial plate are biomechanically superior to all-posterior fixation. And when using a medial plate, the ulnar nerve would be in close contact with it, if not transposed. Therefore, the authors continue to recommend routine ulnar nerve transposition in these fractures.

Outcomes

Results of operative fixation in adult distal humerus fractures have been extensively reported in the literature. Earlier studies recorded 50% to 81% good and excellent clinical results at various institutions [35–40]. Most of these reports stressed rigid anatomic fixation and early motion as the essential aspects of care. More recent studies have documented 84% to 88% good and excellent outcomes with an assortment of outcome measures [41–43].

Others have commented specifically on the functional outcome of patients following these fractures. Gofton and colleagues [44] reported 93% patient satisfaction following open reduction internal fixation of 23 type C distal humerus fractures despite a complication rate of 48%. Elbow motion arc averaged 122°. Aslam and Willett had similar results in their study of 26 patients. In this series, the average motion arc was 112°, with mean pronation of 75° and mean supination of 76°. Although none of the patients were able to regain normal grip strength, 75% of them were able to return to their previous occupation and activities. Also, 85% of these patients reported satisfaction with their outcomes [45]. McKee and colleagues [46] also studied function following internal fixation of distal humerus fractures, using several limb-specific outcome measures. They found most patients to have mild persistent physical impairment, usually caused by range-of-motion and strength deficits in the affected upper extremity. However, general health status, as evaluated by 36-Item Short Form Health Survey (SF-36), was not adversely affected after operative treatment. Finally, Ozdemir and colleagues [47] reported long-term follow-up at an average of 81.5 months following open reduction internal fixation of intra-articular distal humerus fractures. Mean elbow range of motion was from 26° to115°. Predictors of favorable outcomes included closed fractures, boys/men, younger patients, operations using a posterior approach and olecranon osteotomy, and fixation constructs using dual plates.

Authors' preferred method of fixation and technique

At the authors' institution, they have instituted a protocol for complex intra-articular adult distal humerus fractures using parallel plates applied in the sagittal plane. The purpose of using this plate configuration is to maximize distal fragment fixation and stability at the supracondylar level [32].

In approaching a distal humerus fracture, surgical positioning is important for adequate exposure of the surgical site. Surgery may be performed in the prone position, with the arm over a small bump or over the side of the table. This position can sometimes be difficult from an anesthetic standpoint because distal humerus fractures often occur in the elderly. Specifically, these cases can be prolonged, with potential subsequent complications in the prone position.

A somewhat easier approach from an anesthetic and surgical standpoint is to position in the patient supine on the operating table, with a small bump under the scapula on the affected side, which will tend to rotate the upper extremity forward. With hip bolsters on the operative table, the patient can be inclined 20° toward the unaffected side, and the patient can then be draped sterilely, with the arm placed across the chest over a soft bolster. A sterile tourniquet can then be placed high up on the arm to assist with the early surgical exposure of the procedure.

A posterior incision is then made and full thickness skin flaps are created. The ulnar nerve is identified and released in situ for later transposition. In cases involving only the lateral aspect of the distal humerus, the ulnar nerve may not need to be transposed, particularly if an olecranon osteotomy is not going to be performed. In the standard approach to a distal humerus fracture, an osteotomy is performed of the olecranon. The authors prefer an anconeus flap transolecranon approach, which preserves the anconeus innervation and blood supply [28]. Routine osteotomy of the olecranon otherwise tends to denervate the anconeus. Once the anconeus is lifted up as a flap, the osteotomy of the olecranon can be performed (Fig. 4). This procedure can be done as a Chevron-type osteotomy or as a straight osteotomy of the olecranon. The authors prefer a straight osteotomy of the olecranon performed first by use of a sagittal saw to go through the initial posterior cortex of the olecranon.

Next, a wide, flat, sharp osteotome is used to bring the cut approximately half way through the olecranon. This step should be done while visualizing from both the medial and lateral sides to ensure that the osteotomy is being aimed at the center portion of the greater sigmoid notch, which contains minimal cartilage. Once the osteotome has been brought to the half-way mark through the olecranon, the osteotome is levered and the remainder of the olecranon is fractured off from the ulna. This 50% fracture of the olecranon contains interdigitations, which are key to an accurate reduction at the end of the procedure. The olecranon fragment and the anconeus are then retracted proximally, revealing the distal humerus fracture (see Fig. 4).

At this point, the distal humerus fracture is meticulously assembled for fixation. Typically, the distal articular surface, particularly the anterior trochlea and capitellum, are assembled using 2-mm Steinmann pins placed just under the articular surface of the fracture fragment. As these pins are placed, it should be kept in mind that the pins should be kept out of the potential footprint of either a medial or lateral plate for final reduction. Once the distal articular fragments, typically two to three, are reassembled using two to three 2-mm Steinmann pins, they are repositioned onto the end of the humeral shaft, and, using additional pins, they are placed from distal to proximal into the shaft, securing temporary fixation of the distal fragments to the shaft.

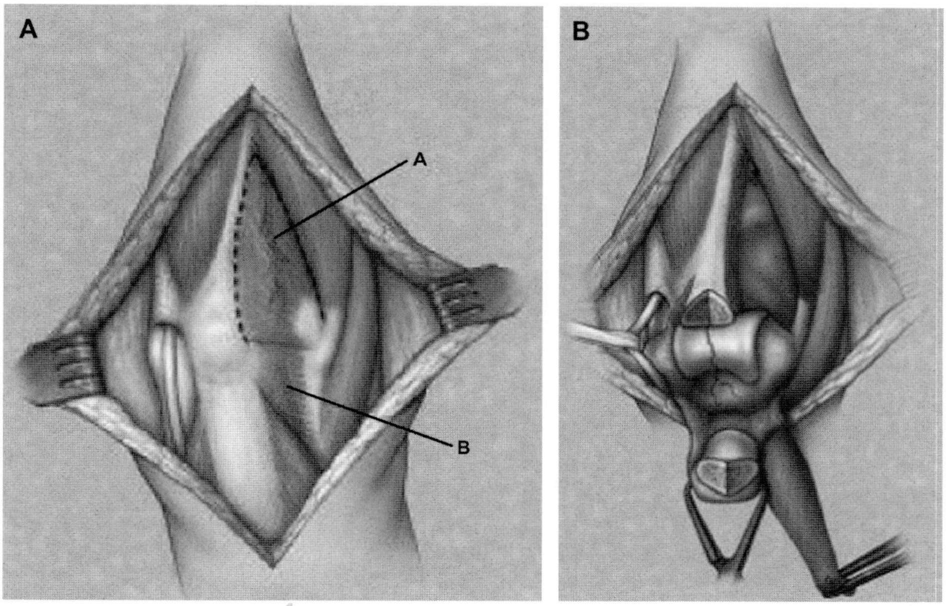

Fig. 4. Anconeus flap transolecranon approach to the distal humerus. (*A*) The anconeus (A) is elevated as a flap to preserve its innervation. (*B*) After the anconeus is elevated, the olecranon (see B in Fig. 4A) osteotomy can be performed in standard fashion. (*From* Athwal GS, Rispoli D, Steinmann SP. The anconeus flap transolecranon approach to the distal humerus; J Orthop Trauma 2006;20(4):282–5; with permission.)

At this point, preliminary fixation of the fracture has been achieved (Fig. 5).

Next, plates are positioned for final fixation. The authors prefer to use precontoured plates for easier application. Additionally, it has been reported that use of such plates is a factor that maximizes fixation [48]. The medial or lateral plate can be applied first, depending on the surgeon's preference. Typically, the plate is reduced to the fracture, held in position with digital pressure, and, using the slotted hole in the plate, preliminary plate fixation is then achieved. The fracture is then inspected and slight readjustments are made, if necessary, through the screw in the oval-slotted hole. When plate fixation seems adequate, a screw is placed on the distal aspect of the plate into the distal fracture construct. At this point, a large bone clamp is used to compress the distal fragment onto the shaft while a compression screw is placed proximally in the plate to achieve good compression of the distal segment to the shaft of the humerus.

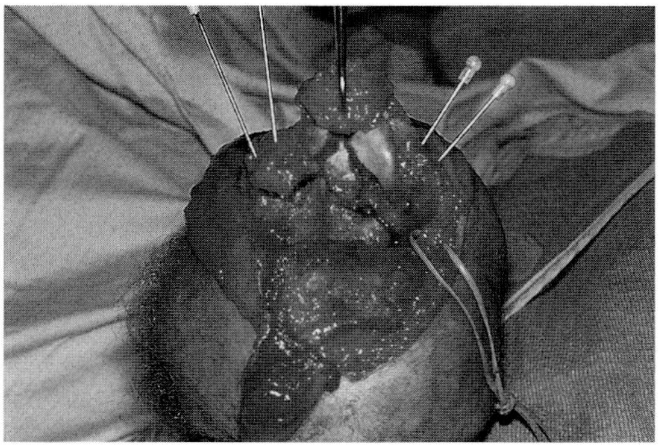

Fig. 5. With significantly comminuted intra-articular fractures, Steinmann pins may be used for provisional fixation.

Likewise, the second plate is placed first with a screw in the slotted hole to allow for adjustment and alignment of the plate. Then a screw is placed into the distal fragment, and, with use of a reduction clamp to compress the distal construct on to the shaft, a compression screw is placed in the proximal aspect of the plate. At this point, further screws are placed into the plates to allow for a strong final construct (Fig. 6). Several companies allow for a locking option in the screws in the proximal and distal aspects of the plates. Particularly in the distal fragment, locking screws allow for a somewhat stronger construct in the softer cancellous bone.

All the screws used in the reduction of the fracture should be placed ideally through the plate

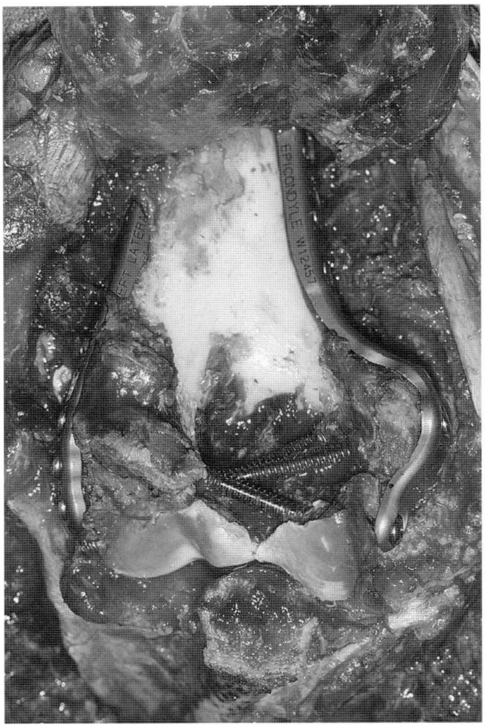

Fig. 6. After the articular surface is reconstructed, pre-contoured parallel plates are applied in the sagittal plane.

to allow greater security and strength of the reduction. Also, the screws should be as long as possible to fix as many fragments as possible in the distal articular construct. Additionally, use of larger 3.5-mm screws, as opposed to smaller 2.7-mm screws, should be used where possible, to strengthen the construct also. Occasionally, screws from a medial and lateral plate will engage each other, which is desirable because it will actually strengthen the construct from the medial to the lateral side (Fig. 7). Once the final screws have been placed into the plates, the elbow joint should be reduced and moved through a full range of motion to identify any evidence of crepitus or catching of the fracture fragments. If noticed, this problem can often be addressed with a bone tamp or a bur to smooth out edges to allow for full motion.

After the articular reduction is checked and found to be adequate, the olecranon osteotomy is reduced to the ulna, and can often be held in place temporarily with a large pin. Plate, screw, or tension-band fixation of the olecranon fragment can then be performed. The authors tend to prefer plate fixation of this fragment because it seems to give greater security to the reduction.

At closure, the ulnar nerve is checked again and transposed into an anterior pouch. A drain is often placed, and staples are typically used in the posterior incision. Postoperatively, the extremity is kept elevated in a sterile dressing, with a posterior plaster splint in the Statue of Liberty position overnight. If strong fixation was felt to be achieved at surgery, immediate active motion can be allowed for the patient. If fixation is inadequate because of significant comminution or osteoporotic bone, motion can be delayed until adequate healing has occurred. The authors prefer this conservative approach in these more tenuous settings because it is easier to address a stiff, healed distal humerus fracture than one which has lost fixation. Additionally, splints and continuous passive motion devices can be used in the post-operative period to help encourage range of motion.

Distal humerus fractures in the elderly

As the proportion and absolute number of distal humerus fractures rise with age, many investigators have begun reporting the results of treatment specifically regarding elderly patients. Although the definition of elderly is certainly open to interpretation, these studies include patients 60 years and older, although many of them focus on older cohorts [49–55]. For example, Srinivasan and colleagues [55] compared nonoperative treatment to open reduction internal fixation in 28 patients with an average age of 85. Operative fixation was found to yield superior results, with a complication rate comparable to that of studies involving younger patients. Several other case series have reported a high rate of good and excellent results comparable to those reported for the population at large (see Refs. [24,49–51, 53,54]).

Other studies reported somewhat less optimistic results, however. Korner and colleagues [52] noted a high complication rate (29%) and only 58% good and excellent results using the Mayo Elbow Performance Score. Although acknowledging the difficulties inherent in treating these often osteoporotic fractures, the investigators nevertheless recommended operative fixation for these injuries in the elderly. Additionally, immobilization times longer than 14 days were discouraged. In contrast, Hausman and Panozzo [49]

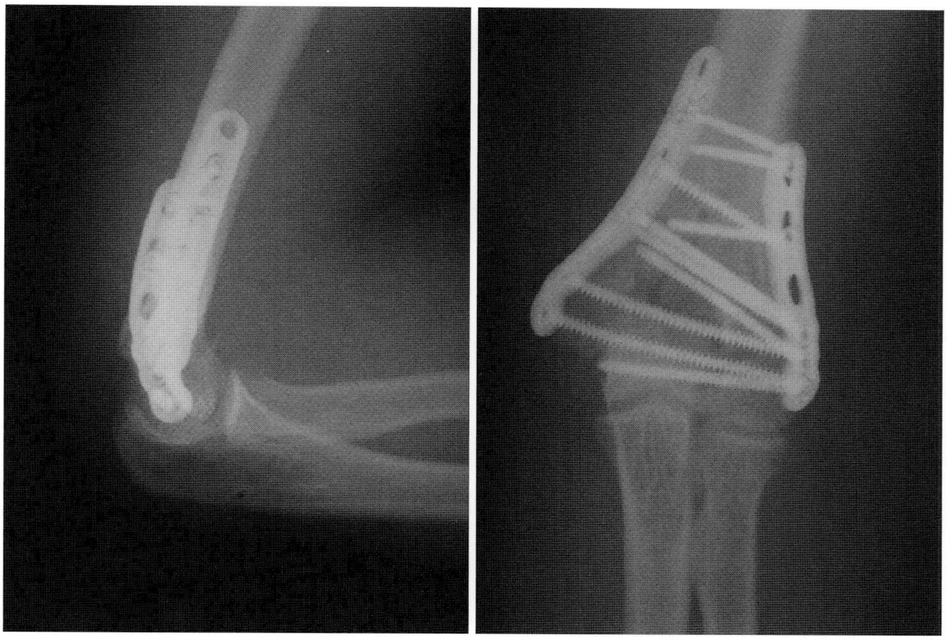

Fig. 7. Use of parallel plating often allows screws to engage each other, resulting in improved fixation. An olecranon osteotomy was not used in this case because the articular surface could be reconstructed without violating the proximal ulna.

recommended postoperative immobilization if fixation is not felt to be sufficiently rigid at the end of surgery. They specifically reference a high rate of success with subsequent contracture release if necessary, but maintain that recovery from lost fixation is less predictable.

Arthroplasty for distal humerus fractures

As TEA emerged as a viable treatment for degenerative disorders of the elbow, many investigators began using this technique in selected, usually elderly, patients and subsequently reporting their results. The first such report, by Cobb and Morrey [56], studied a group of 20 patients (21 elbows) with an average age of 72 treated with primary TEA. They found 100% good and excellent results at an average follow-up of 3.3 years. On the strength of these results, the investigators recommended TEA as a potential alternative in elderly patients. Several other studies have shown satisfactory results with this technique, but long term follow-up is lacking to date [57–63].

Three studies have compared open reduction internal fixation to TEA for treatment of distal humerus fractures in the elderly. Obremskey and colleagues [64] found no strong evidence in support of either treatment modality in an evidence-based review of the literature. Alternatively, Frankle and colleagues [65] reported 100% good and excellent results in women older than 65 with rheumatoid arthritis and other comorbidities treated with TEA. These results compared favorably with the 75% good and excellent results in a more active group treated with internal fixation. TEA was recommended as a viable treatment in these patients, particularly in those with significant comorbidities. Additionally, a recent randomized controlled trial of operative fixation versus TEA in elderly patients who had intra-articular distal humerus fractures found significantly superior Mayo Elbow Performance Scores in the TEA group at 2 years of follow-up [66]. As a result, the authors suggest that TEA is a reasonable treatment alternative for these injuries in select, low-demand, elderly patients, although longer term studies are necessary to define its role fully.

One emerging additional treatment option is hemiarthroplasty for distal humerus fractures (Fig. 8). In this procedure, the medial and lateral columns are reconstructed but the joint surface is left unrepaired. An anatomic distal humerus

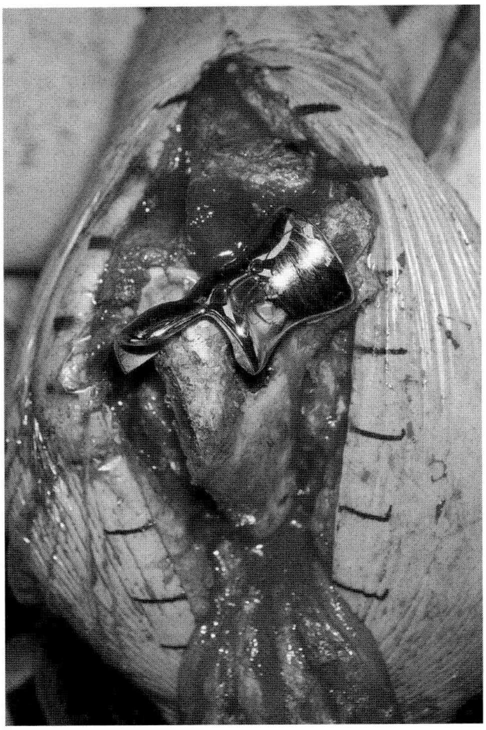

Fig. 8. Distal humeral hemiarthroplasty has been reported with some success in selected patients when the articular surface is not reconstructable.

component from a TEA set is then placed as a substitute to the articular surface. One recent preliminary report of patients treated with Sorbie distal humerus replacement and found all to have good or excellent Mayo Elbow Performance scores (S.P. Steinmann, personal communication).

Complications

Although several clinical studies have reported complication rates with their series, a handful of studies have focused on reporting adverse events following treatment of adult distal humerus fractures. Sodergard and colleagues [67] studied 18 patients who sustained mechanical failure of their fixation constructs. In most of these patients, the cause of failure was unstable fixation, whereas osteoporosis and unknown causes were seen less commonly. The same investigators subsequently reported an average 6-year follow-up study in which 27 of 96 patients suffered postoperative complications. Failure of fixation was the most commonly reported complication (16 patients), but nerve injuries and infections were also seen. Three patients had permanent ulnar nerve dysfunction at final follow-up [68].

Other reports included the aforementioned complications but also noted other problems following operative fixation [69,70]. Kinik and colleagues [69] studied 46 patients treated with open reduction internal fixation. They found nonunion and fixation failure to be relatively uncommon (2%), but reported an approximately 11% rate of nerve complications and significant range of motion loss. Also, 28% of patients were seen to have heterotopic ossification.

Complications of TEA for adult distal humerus fractures are not significantly different from those of TEA for other disorders. Cobb and Morrey [56] noted one fractured ulnar component, three ulnar neuropraxias, and one case of reflex sympathetic dystrophy in their original series. Kamineni and Morrey [60] reported a slightly higher complication rate of 29% in a subsequent series. Although 5 out of 49 elbows required revision surgery, most complications did not require further operative intervention. Other studies reported an overall low rate of complications, with a high rate of clinical success [58,59,61–63].

Summary

Adult distal humerus fractures remain a challenge for the orthopedic surgeon. Additionally, these injuries may be seen with increasing frequency in the future as the proportion of elderly patients in our society continues to rise. Successful treatment and restoration of function are rooted in a firm grasp of the relevant treatment principles. In most patients, internal fixation with modern plates and surgical technique can achieve a satisfactory result. TEA is an alternative treatment in elderly patients who have osteoporotic bone or significant articular comminution not amenable to internal fixation. The role of hemiarthroplasty requires further exploration to delineate its role in these fractures.

References

[1] Robinson CM, H. R., Jacobs N, et al. Adult distal humerus metaphyseal fractures: epidemiology and results of treatment. J Orthop Trauma 2003;17(1):38–47.

[2] Rose SH, M.I.L., Morrey BF, et al. Epidemiologic features of humeral fractures. Clin Orthop Relat Res 1982;168:24–30.

[3] Palvanen M, K. P., Niemi S, et al. Secular trends in the osteoporotic fractures of the distal humerus in elderly women. Eur J Epidemiol 1998;14(2): 159–64.
[4] Muller ME, N. S., Koch P, et al. Comprehensive classification of fractures of long bones. Berlin: Springer-Verlag; 1990.
[5] Jupiter JB, M. D. Fractures of the distal humerus. Orthopedics 1992;15(7):825–33.
[6] Davies MB, S. D. A clinically applicable fracture classification for distal humeral fractures. J Shoulder Elbow Surg 2006;15(5):602–8.
[7] Doornberg J, L. A., Kloen P, et al. Two and three-dimensional computed tomography for the classification and management of distal humeral fractures. J Bone Joint Surg 2006;88(8):1795–801.
[8] Sarmiento A, H. A., Aboulafia A, et al. Functional bracing for comminuted extra-articular fractures of the distal third of the humerus. J Bone Joint Surg Br 1990;72B(2):283–7.
[9] Pehlivan O. Functional treatment of the distal third humeral shaft fractures. Arch Orthop Trauma Surg 2002;122(7):390–5.
[10] Horne G. Supracondylar fractures of the humerus in adults. J Trauma 1980;20(1):71–4.
[11] Niemann K. Condylar fractures of the distal humerus in adults. South Med J 1977;70(8):915–8.
[12] Zagorski JB, J.J., Burkhalter WE, et al. Comminuted intraarticular fractures of the distal humeral condyles. Clin Orthop Relat Res 1986;202: 197–204.
[13] Gabel GT, H.G., Bennett JB, et al. Intraarticular fractures of the distal humerus in the adult. Clin Orthop Relat Res 1987;216:99–108.
[14] Helfet DL, S.G. Bicondylar intraarticular fractures of the distal humerus in adults. Clin Orthop Relat Res 1993;292:26–36.
[15] Imatani J, O. T., Mortio Y, et al. Custom AO small T plate for transcondylar fractures of the distal humerus in the elderly. J Shoulder Elbow Surg 2005; 14(6):611–5.
[16] Zhao J, W. X., Zhang Q. Surgical treatment of comminuted intra-articular fractures of the distal humerus with double tension band osteosynthesis. Orthopedics 2000;23(5):449–52.
[17] Yang KH, P. H., Park SJ, et al. Lateral J-plate fixation in comminuted intercondylar fractures of the humerus. Arch Orthop Trauma Surg 2003;123: 234–8.
[18] Russel GV, J. C., Jones CB, et al. Management of distal humerus fractures with minifragment fixation. J Orthop Trauma 2005;19(7):474–9.
[19] Molloy S, J. L., Burkhart BG, et al. Interference Kirschner wires augment distal humeral fracture fixation in the elderly. J Orthop Trauma 2005; 19(6):377–9.
[20] Levy J, K. S., Hutson JJ, et al. An alternative method of osteosynthesis for distal humeral shaft fractures. J Orthop Trauma 2005;19(1):43–7.
[21] Huang TL, C. F., Chuang TY, et al. Surgical treatment of acute displaced fractures of adult distal humerus with reconstruction plate. Injury 2004;35(11): 1143–8.
[22] Giannoudis PV, A.-L.M., Tzioupis C, et al. Tricortical bone graft for primary reconstruction of comminuted distal humerus fractures. J Orthop Trauma 2005;19(10):741–3.
[23] Self J, V. S., Buford WL Jr, et al. A comparison of double-plate fixation methods for complex distal humerus fractures. J Shoulder Elbow Surg 1995; 4(1):10–6.
[24] Jacobson SR, G. R., Urbaniak JR. Comparison of distal humerus fracture fixation: a biomechanical study. J South Orthop Assoc 1997;6(4):241–9.
[25] Korner J, L. H., Muller LP, et al. The LCP-concept in the operative treatment of distal humerus fractures-biological, biomechanical and surgical aspects. Injury 2003;24:20–30.
[26] Korner J, D. G., Arzdorf M, et al. A biomechanical evaluation of methods of distal humerus fracture fixation using locking compression plates versus conventional reconstruction plates. J Orthop Trauma 2004;18(5):286–93.
[27] Coles CP, B. D., Nork SE, et al. The olecranon osteotomy: a six-year experience in the treatment of intraarticular fractures of the distal humerus. J Orthop Trauma 2006;20(3):164–71.
[28] Athwal GS, R. D., Steinmann SP. The anconeus flap transolecranon approach to the distal humerus. J Orthop Trauma 2006;20(4):282–5.
[29] Ozer H, S. S., Turanli S, et al. Intercondylar fractures of the distal humerus treated with the triceps-reflecting anconeus pedicle approach. Arch Orthop Trauma Surg 2005;125:469–74.
[30] Sanchez-Sotelo J, T. M., O'Driscoll SW. Principle-based internal fixation of distal humerus fractures. Tech Hand Up Extrem Surg 2001;5:179–87.
[31] Ziran BH, S. W., Balk ML, et al. A true triceps-splitting approach for treatment of distal humerus fractures: a preliminary report. J Trauma 2005;58: 70–5.
[32] Sanchez-Sotelo J, T. M., O'Driscoll SW. Complex distal humeral fractures: internal fixation with a principle-based parallel-plate technique. J Bone Joint Surg Am 2007;89-A(5):961–9.
[33] Wang KC, S. H., Hsu KY, et al. Intercondylar fractures of the distal humerus: routine anterior subcutaneous transposition of the ulnar nerve in a posterior operative approach. J Trauma 1994;36(6):770–3.
[34] Gupta R, K. P. Intercondylar fractures of the distal humerus in adults: a critical analysis of 55 cases. Injury 2002;33:511–5.
[35] Caja VL, M. A., Vendemia V, et al. Surgical treatment of bicondylar fractures of the distal humerus. Injury 1994;25(7):433–8.
[36] Holdsworth BJ, M. M. Fractures of the adult distal humerus: elbow function after internal fixation. J Bone Joint Surg Br 1990;72-B(3):362–5.

[37] Jupiter JB, N. U., Holzach P, et al. Intercondylar fractures of the humerus. An operative approach. J Bone Joint Surg Am 1985;67(2):226–39.
[38] Kaushal L, R. J., Singh SP. Comminuted intra-articular fractures of the distal humerus. Int Orthop 1994;18(5):276–9.
[39] Kundel K, B. W., Wieberneit J, et al. Intraarticular distal humerus fractures: factors affecting functional outcome. Clin Orthop Relat Res 1996;332:200–8.
[40] Letsch R, S.-N.K., Sturmer KM, et al. Intraarticular fractures of the distal humerus. Surgical treatment and results. Clin Orthop Relat Res 1989; 241:238–44.
[41] Erlap L, K. M., Sar C, et al. Surgical treatment of distal intraarticular humeral fractures in adults. Int Orthop 2001;25:46–50.
[42] Huang TL, C. F., Chuang TY, et al. The results of open reduction and internal fixation in elderly patients with severe fractures of the distal humerus: a critical analysis of the results. J Trauma 2005; 58(1):62–9.
[43] Soon JL, C. B. Low CO surgical fixation of intra-articular fractures of the distal humerus in adults. Injury 2004;35:44–54.
[44] Gofton WT, M. J., Patterson SD, et al. Functional outcome of AO type C distal humeral fractures. J Hand Surg [Am] 2003;28(2):294–308.
[45] Aslam N, W. K. Functional outcome following internal fixation of intraarticular fractures of the distal humerus (AO type C). Acta Orthop Belg 2004;70(2): 118–22.
[46] McKee MD, W. T., Winston L, et al. Functional outcome following surgical treatment of intra-articular distal humerus fractures through a posterior approach. J Bone Joint Surg Am 2000;82-A(12): 1701–7.
[47] Ozdemir H, U. M., Soyuncu Y, et al. [Long-term functional results of adult intra-articular distal humeral fractures treated by open reduction and plate osteosynthesis]. Acta Orthop Traumatol Turc 2002; 36(4):328–35 [in Turkish].
[48] Waddell JPH, J, Richards R. Supracondylar fractures of the humerus-results of surgical treatment. J Trauma 1988;28(12):1615–21.
[49] Hausman M, P. A. Treatment of distal humerus fractures in the elderly. Clin Orthop Relat Res 2004;425:55–63.
[50] Hubert J, R. R., Neff U, et al. Operative treatment of distal humeral fractures in the elderly. J Bone Joint Surg Br 1994;76-B(5):793–6.
[51] John H, R. R., Neff U, et al. [Distal humerus fractures in patients over 75 years of age. Long-term results of osteosynthesis]. Helv Chir Acta 1993;60(1–2):219–24 [in German].
[52] Korner J, L. H., Muller LP, et al. Distal humerus fractures in elderly patients: results after open reduction and internal fixation. Osteoporos Int 2005;16: S73–9.
[53] Noack W, K.-B.R., Trepte CT. [Indications and results of the surgical treatment of distal intra-articular humeral fractures in the elderly]. Z Orthop Ihre Grenzgeb 1987;125(3):233–42 [in German].
[54] Pereles TR, K. K., Gallagher M, et al. Open reduction and internal fixation of the distal humerus: functional outcome in the elderly. J Trauma 1997;43(4): 578–84.
[55] Srinivasan K, A. M., Matthews SJ, et al. Fractures of the distal humerus in the elderly: is internal fixation the treatment of choice? Clin Orthop Relat Res 2005;434:222–30.
[56] Cobb TK, M. B. Total elbow arthroplasty as primary treatment for distal humeral fractures in elderly patients. J Bone Joint Surg Am 1997;79-A(6):826–32.
[57] Armstrong AD, Y. K. Total elbow arthroplasty and distal humerus elbow fractures. Hand Clin 2004; 20(4):475–83.
[58] Gambirasia R, R. N., Stern R, et al. Total elbow replacement for complex fractures of the distal humerus. An option for the elderly patient. J Bone Joint Surg Br 2001;83-B(7):974–8.
[59] Garcia JA, M. R., Stanley D. Complex fractures of the distal humerus in the elderly. The role of total elbow replacement as primary treatment. J Bone Joint Surg Br 2002;83-B(6):812–6.
[60] Kamineni S, M. B. Distal humeral fractures treated with noncustom total elbow replacement. J Bone Joint Surg Am 2005;87-A(Supp 1, Pt 1): 41–50.
[61] Lee KT, L. C., Singh S. Results of total elbow arthroplasty in the treatment of distal humerus fractures in elderly Asian patients. J Trauma 2006;61(4): 889–92.
[62] Muller LP, K. S., Rommens PM, et al. Primary total elbow replacement for fractures of the distal humerus. Oper Orthop Traumatol 2005;17(2): 119–42.
[63] Ray PS, K. K., Rajsekhar C, et al. Total elbow arthroplasty as primary treatment for distal humeral fractures in elderly patients. Injury 2000;31: 687–92.
[64] Obremskey WT, B. M., Dirschl DR, et al. Internal fixation versus arthroplasty of comminuted fractures of the distal humerus. J Orthop Trauma 2003;17(6):463–5.
[65] Frankle MA, H. D., DiPasquale TG, et al. A comparison of open reduction and internal fixation and primary total elbow arthroplasty in the treatment of intraarticular distal humerus fractures in women older than age 65. J Orthop Trauma 2003;17(7): 473–80.
[66] Veillette CJH, M. M. A multicenter prospective randomized controlled trial of open reduction internal fixation versus total elbow arthroplasty for displaced intra-articular distal humeral fractures

in elderly patients. J Shoulder Elbow Surg 2007; 16(2):e52.

[67] Sodergard J, S. J., Bostman O. Mechanical failures of internal fixation in T and Y fractures of the distal humerus. J Trauma 1992;33(5): 687–90.

[68] Sodergard J, S. J., Bostman O. Postoperative complications of distal humeral fractures. 27/96 adults followed up for 6 (2–10) years. Acta Orthop Scand 1992;63(1):85–9.

[69] Kinik J, A. H., Mergen E. Management of distal humerus fractures in adults. Arch Orthop Trauma Surg 1999;119:467–9.

[70] Ring D, J. J. Complex fractures of the distal humerus and their complications. J Shoulder Elbow Surg 1999;8(1):85–97.

ELSEVIER
SAUNDERS

Hand Clin 23 (2007) 471–479

HAND
CLINICS

Apparent Capitellar Fractures

David Ring, MD, PhD

Hand and Upper Extremity Service, Orthopaedic Trauma Service, Department of Orthopaedic Surgery, Massachusetts General Hospital, Yawkey 2100, 55 Fruit Street, Boston, MA 02114, USA

In 1996, McKee and colleagues [1] emphasized that many capitellum fractures extend into the trochlea, but this was not a new finding. In fact, it has been identified in a large percentage of published case series for nearly a century [2–11]. More recent series have consistently identified even greater complexity, with frequent fracture of the lateral epicondyle, impaction of the posterolateral aspect of the humerus and the trochlea, fragmentation of the articular surface, and even involvement of the medial epicondyle (Fig. 1).

It has been difficult to decide how best to label or describe these fractures. One recent series refers to them as capitellar and trochlear fractures [12]. Two others refer to them as articular fractures of the distal humerus [13,14]. I have come to prefer a more practical label: "apparent capitellar fractures." My reasoning is that most orthopaedic surgeons perceive these fractures as capitellar fractures, even though recent series consistently emphasize that isolated capitellar fractures are uncommon [12–14]. It's not surprising that most surgeons would identify these fractures as isolated fractures of the capitellum, even when they are more complex, because the displaced capitellar fracture fragment is usually the most obvious and identifiable radiographic finding, and because teaching has traditionally underemphasized the frequent involvement of the trochlea and the potential for greater complexity with these fractures.

The label "apparent capitellar fracture" is practical because it emphasizes the need to look more closely. In particular, radiographs are rarely sufficient to characterize these lesions, and three-dimensional CT (3DCT) reconstructions with the radius and ulna subtracted are invaluable for preoperative planning. As complex as many of these fractures are, three recent studies have found that operative repair is successful at maintaining the native elbow, with satisfactory function in most patients. As a salvage procedure, or in very complex acute fractures (particularly in low-demand, infirm patients, or those with prior articular damage), the absence of columnar involvement makes distal humeral hemiarthroplasty an appealing treatment option.

Relevant anatomy

The elbow is an inherently stable joint. The nearly 180 capture of the trochlea in the trochlear notch is tilted somewhat posterior, thereby increasing the anterior buttress of the coronoid process [15]. The trochlea is wide and has a central groove that interdigitates with a ridge in the center of the trochlear notch. The contacts between (1) the anteromedial coronoid facet and the medial lip of the trochlea and (2) the radial head and capitellum represent the most important stabilizing columns of the elbow. In the absence of a radial head or capitellum, the contact between the lateral lip of the trochlea and the lateral portion of the coronoid becomes more important.

The trochlea is supported by medial and lateral columns of bone, with the central area of the distal humerus (the olecranon and coronoid fossae) being relatively devoid of bone. The lateral column curves anteriorly along with the anteriorly translated articular surface of the distal humerus, but the medial column is straight, in line with the humeral diaphysis. A plate placed on the lateral surface of the distal humerus should therefore curve anterior distally; a straight plate may risk fixing the distal humerus in a relatively straight position, which can restrict flexion.

E-mail address: dring@partners.org

0749-0712/07/$ - see front matter
doi:10.1016/j.hcl.2007.09.004

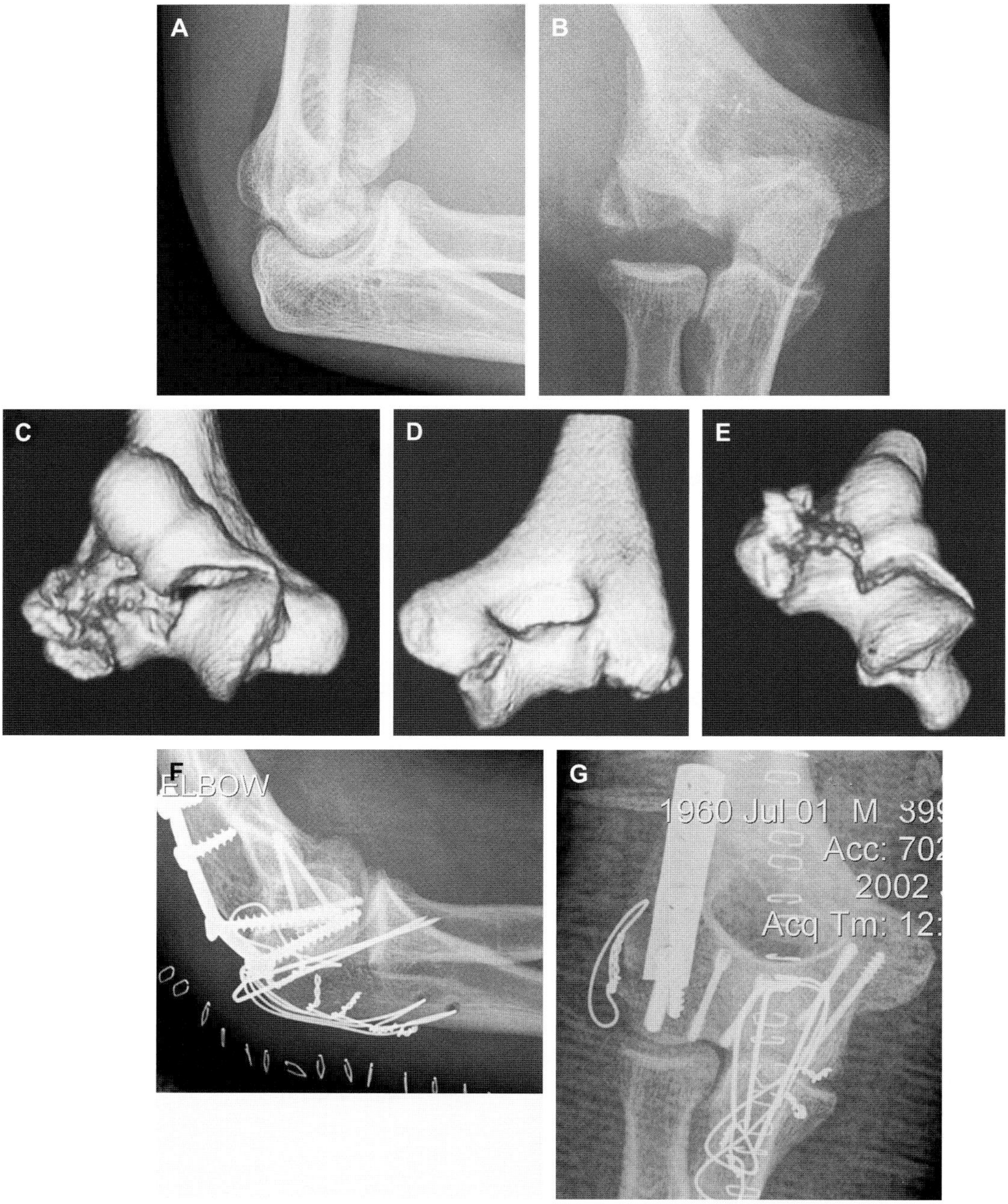

Fig. 1. Apparent capitellum fractures are often more than they seem. (*A*) Lateral radiograph demonstrates the presence of two "arcs" on the fragment that is displaced anterior and proximal. This so-called "double-arc sign" indicates that the fracture extends well into the capitellum. (*B*) On the anteroposterior view, it is apparent in this case that more than the capitellum is involved. (*C*) Three-dimensional CT shows the true extent of the fracture. With the radius and ulna subtracted, it is apparent that there is a large anterior capitellum and trochlear fragment, but also that there is an impacted (stable) fracture of the posterior trochlea. (*D*) Posterior three-dimensional CT view shows the fracture line and impaction of the trochlea and the posterior aspect of the lateral column. (*E*) Inferior view shows this even better. (*F*) Lateral view after operative fixation with many buried screws and a posterolateral plate. (*G*) Anteroposterior view shows the headless buried screws.

Elbow implants must respect articular surfaces, fossae, and neurovascular structures. Transposition of the ulnar nerve provides additional nonarticular sites for fixation of the medial column of the distal humerus and the medial aspect of the coronoid process. The lateral aspect of the posterior column is nonarticular (ie, the capitellum is an anterior structure) and can accommodate a plate to the distal limit of the humerus. The radial nerve is relatively safe unless a very proximal exposure of the humeral diaphysis is needed, or a hinged external fixator is applied, in which case care should be taken to protect the nerve as it crosses from posterior to anterior on the lateral aspect of the humerus.

Classification

Capitellum fractures have long been classified as (1) a thick fragment, (2) a thin fragment, or (3) a comminuted fragment [16]. Most likely, many of the more complex fractures went unrecognized, and others were considered among the "comminuted" fractures. It is remarkable and humbling, but humans cannot see what they don't understand or recognize. It may be that, in the current era of increasing subspecialization, some surgeons are getting an opportunity to operate on a few of these uncommon fractures each year, rather than a few in their entire career, as was the likely situation in the past. This theory as to why these fracture characteristics and patterns were underappreciated in the past is plausible but speculative. Improved diagnostic and operative technique likely also played a role.

The injury seems to progress, with any fracture involving more than the anterior surface of the capitellum and trochlea also creating a fracture of the lateral epicondyle, followed by the next stage of impaction of the lateral column of the distal humerus, then fracture of the posterior aspect of the trochlea, and finally, fracture of the medial epicondyle [13]. Dubberly and colleagues [12] classified fractures as involving the capitellum with or without a small part of the lateral trochlear ridge (type 1), the capitellum and the trochlea as one large fragment (type 2), and the capitellum and trochlear with fragmentation (type 3). Each type is subclassified according to the presence (subtype B) or absence (subtype A) of posterior fracture. The importance of identifying fractures of the posterior aspect of the distal humerus was emphasized in all three recent series [12–14].

Evaluation

The complexity of the fracture is usually not readily apparent on standard radiographs. The so-called "double arc" sign indicates that a substantial portion of the trochlea is on the anteriorly and proximally displaced fracture fragment (see Fig. 1) [1]. The ulnohumeral joint often appears incongruent on the lateral view because the ulna settles into the defect in the humerus. With careful examination, it may be possible to see a trochlear defect on the anteroposterior view. Radiographs cannot demonstrate impaction (stable malalignment of fracture fragments) or fragmentation.

Two-dimensional CT images depict fracture detail, but can be difficult to interpret, particularly if there is any obliquity in the scan plane. I find 3DCT to be much more intuitive and straightforward to interpret. The radius and ulna need to be extracted from the images to see the articular surface of the distal humerus well. In my experience, 3DCT scans with surface rendering accurately depict the number and location of fracture fragments, fracture impaction, and epicondylar/columnar involvement. The detailed understanding of the fracture pattern provided by 3DCT allows for thorough and accurate preoperative planning (see Fig. 1).

We studied the influence of 3DCT on classification of fractures, identification of important fracture characteristics, and management decisions [17]. The improvement in intraobserver reliability supports the contention that the scans are easier to interpret. It's unclear how to interpret the lack of improvement in agreement between different observers (interobserver) reliability, but I think it reflects variations in experience and understanding, more than shortcomings of the imaging techniques.

Recently, we have done pilot work with three-dimensional models created from CT scan data (Fig. 2) [18]. (Medical Modeling LLC, Golden, Colorado), which may add an additional level of visuospatial understanding of the fracture and may also allow for additional planning and perhaps even a preoperative "practice run" using the models.

Treatment options

Closed reduction and cast immobilization has been used with some reported success in the past [19]; however, given that most apparent capitellum fractures involve the lateral trochlea, this

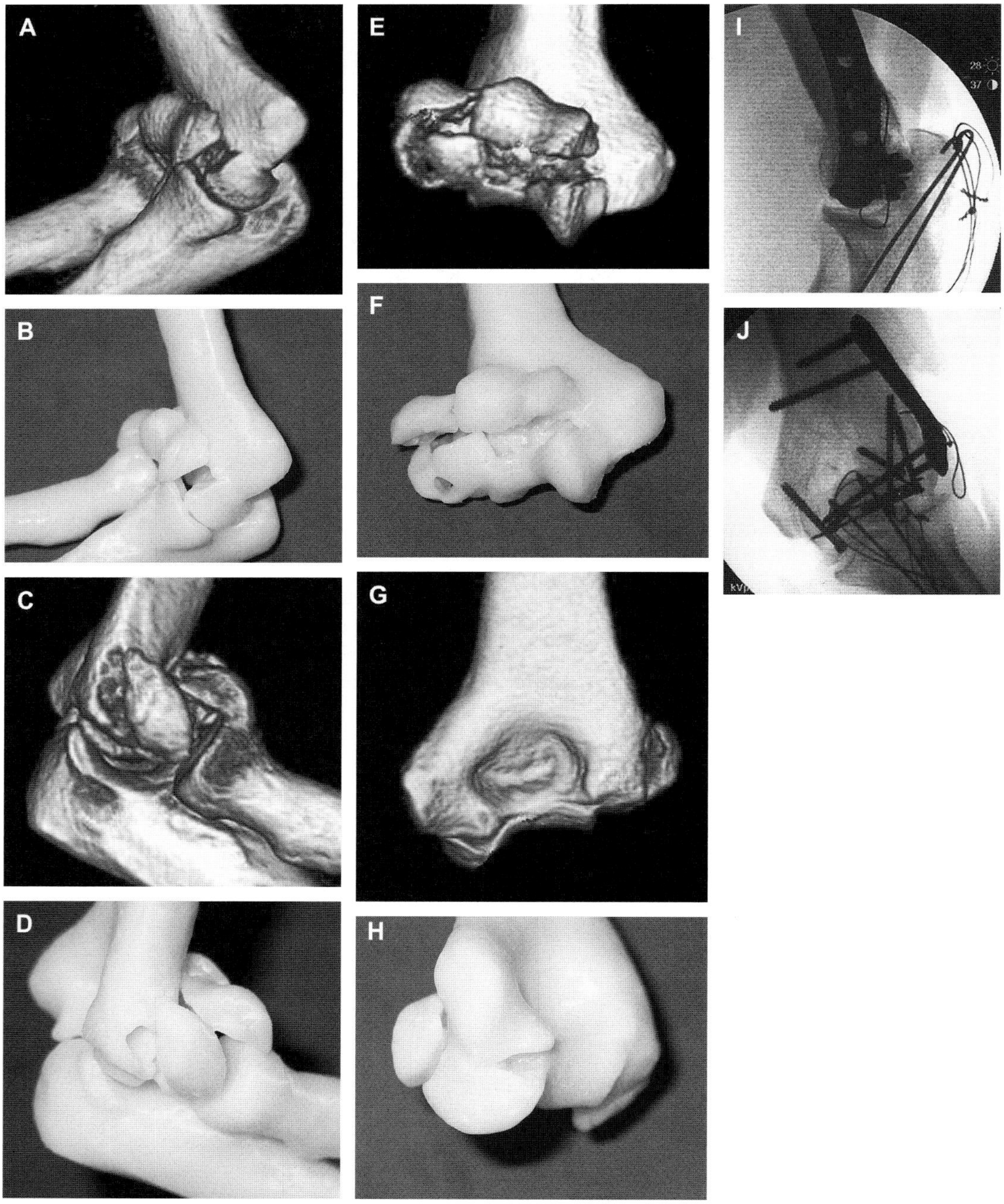

Fig. 2. Three-dimensional CT and three-dimensional models can greatly facilitate the surgeon's understanding of the fracture, which helps plan and execute internal fixation. (*A*) Medial view 3DCT. (*B*) Medial view of model. (*C*) Lateral view 3DCT. (*D*) Lateral view of model. (*E*) Anterior view 3DCT. (*F*) Anterior view of model. (*G*) Posterior view 3DCT. (*H*) Posteromedial view of model. (*I*) Intraoperative lateral image shows near anatomic fixation with small buried wires and headless screws and a lateral plate. (*Courtesy of* Acumed, Beaverton, Oregon, with permission.) (*J*) Intraoperative anteroposterior image shows the same.

approach risks malunion, which may restrict motion and contribute to arthrosis. Excision of the fragments, which also has supporters [19], has similar disadvantages. I would only consider nonoperative treatment or fragment excision in infirm, low-demand patients.

Prosthetic elbow arthroplasty is considered when the fracture is so complex that some important fragments cannot be repaired, or in the presence of pre-existing articular degeneration (eg, rheumatoid arthritis). Because most apparent capitellar fractures do not involve the medial and lateral columns, it is possible to consider distal humeral hemiarthroplasty, although this should still be considered experimental. Total elbow arthroplasty has been associated with good short-term results [20,21], but there is concern about long-term performance. Elbow prostheses loosen with time, and strict activity restrictions (5 kg lifting limit) are recommended for maximal longevity. Another concern is that infection is more common with prosthetic arthroplasty in the elbow than in the knee or hip, and more difficult to salvage.

In contrast, successful open reduction and internal fixation will restore the native elbow. Despite some degree of impairment from stiffness and articular injury, a functioning native elbow is allowed unlimited activity. Fixation of complex fractures with several entirely, or nearly entirely, articular fracture fragments can be challenging. It is more important for the patient to be treated by a surgeon who is familiar with these fractures and how to repair them than it is for the patient to be treated promptly. Patients who are treated with splinting, pain medication, and frequent hand exercise to limit swelling can wait 2 or 3 weeks for definitive surgery, if necessary.

Preoperative planning

It is useful to have headless screws, small threaded Kirschner wires, and plates with relatively small distal screws (2.0–2.7 mm) to facilitate internal fixation. If 3DCT confirms that the fracture extends to involve the posterior aspect of the trochlea or the medial epicondyle, then an olecranon osteotomy may provide better exposure for reduction and internal fixation than an extended lateral exposure, which is satisfactory in most cases. Distal humeral hemiarthroplasty can be performed through an olecranon osteotomy, but total elbow arthroplasty is more difficult in the presence of an osteotomy. If the surgeon anticipates that prosthetic arthroplasty may be necessary based on 3DCT, the prosthesis should be available and the operative exposure should be modified as needed.

Operative techniques

Operative exposure

An extended lateral exposure can be used for most complex articular fractures, but if the posterior aspect of the trochlea and the medial epicondyle are fractured, an olecranon osteotomy is preferable. When using an olecranon osteotomy, it is usually necessary to mobilize the lateral epicondyle fracture (which has the origins of the lateral collateral ligament and the common wrist and digit extensors) and externally rotate the humerus away from the coronoid and radial head, thereby improving anterior exposure. This procedure allows for retrieval of the anterior capitellum and trochlear fragments, which are often dislocated anteriorly and proximally out of the trochlear notch of the ulna. If the surgeon is considering a total elbow arthroplasty (eg, in the setting of severe pre-existing articular damage), then an olecranon osteotomy should not be used; however, an olecranon osteotomy provides good exposure for a distal humerus hemiarthroplasty.

Operative technique: extensile lateral exposure

A midline posterior or a lateral skin incision can be used. The patient is positioned supine, with the arm supported on a hand table. A sterile pneumatic tourniquet is used. When the lateral epicondyle is fractured, it can be mobilized and retracted distally along with the attached origins of the wrist and digital extensor muscles and the lateral collateral ligament complex; otherwise, the lateral collateral ligament may need to be released (either directly or by way of osteotomy) for exposure.

The more proximal origins of the radial wrist extensor muscles are elevated from the lateral supracondylar ridge to improve the exposure to the anterior articular fragments. The exposure is completed by the elevation of the lateral aspect of the triceps from the distal humerus and the proximal olecranon, permitting the elbow joint to be hinged open, thereby providing exposure to the anterior and posterior articular surfaces of the distally humerus.

Operative technique: olecranon osteotomy

The patient is placed in a lateral decubitus position, with the arm supported over a bolster. Either the prior incision or a straight posterior incision is used. Medial and lateral skin flaps are elevated, with care taken to protect cutaneous nerve branches and keep them within the skin flaps. The ulnar nerve is identified along the medial border of the triceps, dissected at least 6 cm proximally and distally, and left in an anteriorly transposed position in the subcutaneous tissues.

The insertion of the anconeus onto the proximal ulna is partially elevated to view the arc of the trochlear notch directly. Alternatively, if the ulnar nerve has been transposed, the medial elbow capsule can be incised in the bed where the ulnar nerve originally lay. If the fracture is simple enough that reduction of the metaphyseal fracture lines can be relied on to achieve a good articular reduction, the triceps can be elevated from the posterior aspect of the distal humerus on the medial and lateral sides, and the osteotomy made only if necessary. In most patients, however, an osteotomy is necessary for adequate reduction and fixation.

An apex distal chevron-shaped osteotomy is planned so that it enters the joint at the depths of the trochlear notch. An oscillating saw is used to start the osteotomy. A small straight osteotome is then used to complete it, by levering the osteotome proximally and cracking the subchondral bone. This maneuver creates an uneven surface that facilitates repositioning and may enhance stability. The posterior elbow capsule is then incised and the olecranon fragment and triceps are elevated from the posterior aspect of the humerus.

Many techniques for internal fixation of the osteotomy have been described, including screws, tension-band wiring techniques, and plate and screw fixation. I prefer to use two parallel 0.045-in Kirschner wires drilled obliquely across the osteotomy site so that they engage the anterior ulnar cortex distal to the coronoid process, and two 22-gauge stainless steel figure-of-eight tension-band wires, using a technique described elsewhere [22].

Fixation techniques

A fracture involving the capitellum and trochlea usually can only be realigned and secured without taking down the lateral collateral ligament complex. The metaphyseal fracture lines are realigned, the fracture is held provisionally with Kirschner wires, and then the fracture is secured with headless countersunk screws or screws entering from the posterior, nonarticular portion of the lateral column. More complex fractures nearly always involve a fracture of the lateral epicondyle. Mobilization of the epicondyle with the attached common extensors and lateral collateral ligament origin provides excellent exposure of the anterior articular surface.

Apparent capitellum fractures consist primarily of entirely articular fragments that can only be secured with implants that are countersunk beneath the articular surface (see Fig. 2) [13,23]. Small threaded Kirschner wires can be useful in this regard because there is often limited bone opposite these fragments for internal fixation. The small threaded Kirschner wires can be placed through the edge of the fracture site connecting the subchondral bone of adjacent fragments. When the major articular fragments are reduced, the small wires are buried. For larger articular fragments with an opposite bony support, headless screws (the Herbert screw and variations, many of which are now cannulated) are useful. I would caution against the use of countersunk threaded screws because these allow settling, which results in protrusion of the screw head into the joint; it's better if the head is threaded so that it cannot back out as easily. Many of the newer custom plates for the distal humerus incorporate small distal screws that can be aligned along the subchondral bone of the articular fragment. Some of these screws can lock to the plate if this seems advantageous, which is most often the case in poor quality bone. The lateral epicondyle is usually a very small fragment; it can be secured with either a plate or small tension wires that engage the soft tissue attachments.

When the anterior articular fracture fragments don't fit into the fracture bed, there is usually posterior impaction of the posterior aspect of the lateral column with or without impaction of the posterior trochlea (see Fig. 2). This impaction must be pushed back into place to achieve reduction. Impaction, meaning that the articular fragments are fractured but are pushed into the bone, settling into a relatively stable position that might not be perceived as fractured, is increasingly recognized in articular fractures of the upper extremity. Anticipation and recognition of impaction will facilitate reduction and fixation.

Elbow arthroplasty

For complex columnar fractures involving the medial and lateral columns of the distal humerus, elbow arthroplasty must be linked to account for the loss of the epicondyles and therefore the stability provided by the collateral ligaments. The increasing use of total elbow arthroplasty for the treatment of complex fractures of the distal humerus [20,24–26] reflects surgeon dissatisfaction with open reduction and internal fixation in many cases. This approach became possible after the development of successful, semiconstrained elbow arthroplasties that do not require the retention of collateral ligaments or other stabilizing structures. As a result, total elbow arthroplasty for fracture is one of the easiest types of total elbow arthroplasties to perform because the prosthesis can be inserted without releasing the triceps from the proximal ulna, by working in the space created by resecting the distal fracture fragments, including the medial and lateral epicondyles [25].

The rapid recovery and excellent early results also increase the appeal of total elbow arthroplasty for fractures of the distal humerus [20]. I believe that the results are seductively good, because the surgeon will gladly abandon tedious and challenging attempts to repair a complex distal humerus fracture and celebrate his or her decision by virtue of the more rapid return to function; however, the patient will now have to limit use of the limb severely, prepare for the eventual failure of the prosthesis, and occasionally experience a severe complication, such as a wound dehiscence or deep infection, which are much more difficult to treat after total elbow arthroplasty than after internal fixation.

For total elbow arthroplasty, the ulnar nerve is completely released and transposed anteriorly into the subcutaneous tissues. The fracture fragments, including the medial and lateral epicondyles, are excised and the triceps is elevated from the posterior aspect of the humerus. The triceps is elevated slightly from the olecranon tip that will be excised to facilitate passage of the ulnar component of the prosthesis, but there is no need for an extensive elevation of the triceps from the ulna in the treatment of a distal humerus fracture with total elbow arthroplasty; a sufficient working space is created by removing the fracture fragments.

A semiconstrained (linked) total elbow arthroplasty is inserted according to the specific technique for the implant used. Repair of the common extensor and flexor muscles can improve coverage of the implant, but is not necessary for good arm function. The elbow is splinted for comfort only, and the patient is allowed to begin active use and exercise of the arm as soon as he or she is able.

A hemiarthroplasty can be inserted through an olecranon osteotomy. Insertion of the prosthesis is relatively straightforward after excision of any remaining articular fragments. In fact, it may be necessary to provide some support for the prosthesis with extra methyl methacrylate cement. An unlinked prosthesis with a relatively anatomic shape is necessary. The humeral component of the Sorbie elbow prosthesis (Wright Medical, Memphis, Tennessee) is well suited to this. Another option is the Latitude prosthesis (Tournier Eden Prairie, Minnesota).

Rehabilitation

The elbow is prone to stiffness with prolonged immobilization, and the goal of treatment is secure fixation allowing immediate elbow mobilization. On the other hand, a healed, well-aligned fracture takes precedence, particularly with complex fractures, because capsular contracture can be addressed with subsequent surgery if needed, but early loss of fixation or articular damage may be irrecoverable.

The hand is typically swollen and ecchymotic after an elbow injury and can become permanently stiff if confident active exercises are not encouraged. Active exercises and gentle functional use of the arm for daily activities is usually initiated within a few days, most often starting the morning after surgery, but that may be delayed for as long as a month if the fixation is relatively tenuous. The patient is encouraged to use his or her other hand, gravity, and pushing against other objects to help assist with elbow mobilization. Useful tools for increasing motion include either static progressive (a position of static stretch is applied and adjusted as the pain dissipates) or dynamic (a constant dynamic force is applied to the elbow) elbow splints.

The use of continuous passive elbow motion (using various devices), with or without continuous anesthesia, by way of a brachial plexus catheter, is gaining popularity despite the lack of evidence that it improves elbow motion. It is not clear that the additional risk and cost are justified. I believe that active elbow motion is the key and that motivated patients will do better; I therefore shy away from passive treatments.

Passive manipulation by a therapist or family member is discouraged because it is believed that this will contribute to heterotopic bone formation. It may also loosen implants or impede healing. In addition, the patient must learn how to mobilize his or her own arm if the exercise program is to be effective.

Complications

Ulnar neuropathy

Ulnar neuropathy can develop after treatment of apparent capitellum fractures, even when an extended lateral exposure is used. The ulnar nerve is vulnerable to constriction as it runs through the cubital tunnel fascia and Osborne's fascia, particularly in the setting of posttraumatic swelling, bleeding, tissue injury and distortion, scar formation and tissue contracture, heterotopic ossification, and arthrosis. When it occurs, ulnar nerve dysfunction can contribute to stiffness and pain, and can affect hand function [27]. It is important to be aware of the importance of the ulnar nerve, and always evaluate for symptoms and signs of ulnar nerve dysfunction, being particularly suspicious when stiffness or pain are greater than might otherwise be expected. Because it is difficult to detect ulnar neuropathy during recovery from an apparent capitellum fracture, some consideration has been given to routine in situ ulnar nerve decompression [28].

Ulnar nerve dysfunction can result from entrapment by normal anatomic structures or scar, but can also result from handling and transposition of the nerve. It can be difficult to predict when the nerve will have dysfunction after transposition, but vigorous retraction seems to be the most preventable aspect of treatment; for this reason, I use a small vessel loop rather than a Penrose drain to isolate the nerve and assist with dissection and I never attach a clamp to the loop. It is also useful to have an oscillating drill to avoid wrapping the nerve up on the drill.

Acute ulnar nerve dysfunction with an intact nerve (either due to the injury or handling of the nerve during surgery) usually, but not always, recovers. In can take a long time, in some cases more than a year or more, to recover. Serial clinical examination and nerve conduction studies and electromyography can help determine if surgical intervention is worthwhile. Operative treatment is considered if serial neurophysiologic testing does not demonstrate improvement, or if examination indicates obvious worsening of the deficit.

Stiffness and heterotopic ossification

Failure to restore the anterior translation of the trochlea with respect to the humeral shaft will lead to limitation of flexion that cannot be improved with capsular release. Articular incongruities and arthrosis can also result in unsalvageable stiffness. Heterotopic ossification that blocks motion usually occurs on the anterior aspect of the distal humerus after distal humerus fracture, causing limitation of flexion. Resection of this bone is straightforward, restores flexion, and does not required prophylaxis against recurrence because recurrence after resection of this anterior heterotopic bone is unusual.

Nonunion and osteonecrosis

Nonunion of entirely articular fragments is unusual. It is most common in the setting of osteonecrosis, in which case the fragments must be excised. It is surprising how uncommon osteonecrosis occurs, given that many of the fragments have no blood supply. Furthermore, the lateral trochlea does not seem to be as susceptible to osteonecrosis as are the capitellar fragments. Larger, viable articular fragments can be treated with open reduction in internal fixation and autogenous cancellous bone grafting [29]. Total elbow arthroplasty can also be used to salvage nonunion of the distal humerus, but is most appropriate in older, low-demand patients [30,31]. Total elbow arthroplasty for posttraumatic reconstruction may have an increased rate of complications [32].

Infection

Fortunately, infections are very uncommon after the operative treatment of elbow fractures. They are usually related to complex open injuries and devitalized fracture fragments, and usually affect immunocompromised patients. These infections are often treated with serial debridement, retention of implants, and parenteral antibiotics, particularly when the fracture is complex. Healing of the fractures can usually be achieved with this regimen. Eventually, complete eradication of the infection usually requires implant removal. Unfortunately, this approach may be less successful with apparent capitellar fractures because many of the fracture fragments have no blood supply.

References

[1] McKee MD, Jupiter JB, Bamberger HB. Coronal shear fractures of the distal end of the humerus. J Bone Joint Surg Am 1996;78A:49–54.

[2] Mazel MS. Fracture of the capitellum: a report of a case. J Bone Joint Surg Am 1935;17:483–8.

[3] Fowles JV, Kassab MT. Fracture of the capitulum humeri: treatment by excision. J Bone Joint Surg Am 1974;56A:794–8.

[4] Grantham SA, Norris TR, Bush DC. Isolated fracture of the humeral capitellum. Clin Orthop Relat Res 1981;161:262–9.

[5] Collert S. Surgical management of fracture of the capitulum humeri. Arch Orthop Scand 1977;48:603–6.

[6] Darrach W. Fracture of lower articular surface of humerus. Ann Surg 1916;64:724–5.

[7] Lindem MC. Fractures of the capitellum and trochlea. Ann Surg 1922;76:78–82.

[8] Lee WE, Summey TJ. Fracture of the capitellum of the humerus. Ann Surg 1934;99:497–509.

[9] Oppenheim W, Davlin LB, Leipzig JM, et al. Concomitant fractures of the capitellum and trochlea. J Orthop Trauma 1989;3:260–2.

[10] Rhodin R. On the treatment of fracture of the capitellum. Acta Chir Scand 1942;86:475–86.

[11] Gejrot W. On intra-articular fractures of the capitellum and trochlea of the humerus with special reference to the treatment. Acta Chir Scand 1932;71:253–70.

[12] Dubberley JH, Faber KJ, Macdermid JC, et al. Outcome after open reduction and internal fixation of capitellar and trochlear fractures. J Bone Joint Surg Am 2006;88(1):46–54.

[13] Ring D, Gulotta L, Jupiter J. Articular fractures of the distal part of the humerus. J Bone Joint Surg Am 2003;85A:232–8.

[14] Watts AC, Morris A, Robinson CM. Fractures of the distal humeral articular surface. J Bone Joint Surg Br 2007;89(4):510–5.

[15] Kapandji IA. The physiology of the joints. 5th edition. Edinburgh (UK): Churchill Livingstone; 1982.

[16] Bryan RS, Morrey BF. Fractures of the distal humerus. In: Morrey BF, editor. The elbow and its disorders. Philadelphia: WB Saunders; 1985. p. 302–39.

[17] Doornberg J, Lindenhovius A, Kloen P, et al. Two and three-dimensional computed tomography for the classification and management of distal humeral fractures. Evaluation of reliability and diagnostic accuracy. J Bone Joint Surg Am 2006; 88(8):1795–801.

[18] Jupiter JB, Ruder J, Roth DA. Computer-generated bone models in the planning of osteotomy of multidirectional distal radius malunions. J Hand Surg [Am] 1992;17(3):406–15.

[19] Dushuttle RP, Coyle MP, Zawadsky JP, et al. Fractures of the capitellum. J Trauma 1985;25(4): 317–21.

[20] Frankle MA, Herscovici D, Pasquale TF, et al. A comparison of open reduction and internal fixation and primary total elbow arthroplasty in the treatment of intraarticular distal humerus fractures in women older than age 65. J Orthop Trauma 2003;17:473–80.

[21] Kamineni S, Morrey BF. Distal humeral fractures treated with noncustom total elbow replacement. J Bone Joint Surg Am 2004;86-A(5):940–7.

[22] Ring D, Gulotta L, Chin K, et al. Olecranon osteotomy for exposure of fractures and nonunions of the distal humerus. J Orthop Trauma 2004; 18(7):446–9.

[23] Jupiter JB, Barnes KA, Goodman LJ, et al. Multiplane fracture of the distal humerus. J Orthop Trauma 1993;7:216–20.

[24] Garcia JA, Mykula R, Stanley D. Complex fractures of the distal humerus in the elderly. The role of total elbow replacement as primary treatment. J Bone Joint Surg Br 2001;84B:812–6.

[25] Cobb TK, Morrey BF. Total elbow arthroplasty as primary treatment for distal humerus fractures in elderly patients. J Bone Joint Surg Am 1997;79A: 826–32.

[26] Ray PS, Kakarlapudi K, Rajsekhar C, et al. Total elbow arthroplasty as primary treatment for distal humeral fractures in elderly patients. Injury 2000;31: 687–92.

[27] Faierman E, Wang J, Jupiter JB. Secondary ulnar nerve palsy in adults after elbow trauma: a report of two cases. J Hand Surg [Am] 2001;26A:675–8.

[28] Shin R, Ring D. The ulnar nerve in elbow trauma. J Bone Joint Surg Am 2007;89(5):1108–16.

[29] Ring D, Jupiter JB. Operative treatment of osteochondral nonunion of the distal humerus. J Orthop Trauma 2006;20(1):56–9.

[30] Morrey BF, Adams RA. Semiconstrained elbow replacement for distal humeral nonunion. J Bone Joint Surg Br 1995;77B:67–72.

[31] Figgie MP, Inglis AE, Mow CS, et al. Salvage of non-union of supracondylar fracture of the humerus by total elbow arthroplasty. J Bone Joint Surg Am 1989;71A:1058–65.

[32] Hildebrand KA, Patterson SD, Regan WD, et al. Functional outcome of semiconstrained total elbow arthroplasty. J Bone Joint Surg Am 2000;82A: 1379–86.

ELSEVIER
SAUNDERS

Hand Clin 23 (2007) 481–486

HAND
CLINICS

Fractures of the Capitellum

Emilie V. Cheung, MD

Department of Orthopedic Surgery, Stanford University, 300 Pasteur Drive, Edwards R-155, MC 5335, Stanford, CA 94305, USA

The capitellum forms the anterior and inferior articular surface of the distal humerus as a smooth, round, hemispheric structure. Its articular surface does not extend posterior to the coronal plane of the humeral face. Fractures of the capitellum are rare injuries, and account for less than 1% of all elbow fractures [1,2]. Most series have a female predominance [3–9], which has been thought to be associated with cubitus valgus, cubitus recurvatum, or osteoporosis [5,9].

The mechanism of injury is usually a fall onto the outstretched hand, with the elbow partially flexed or extended. An axial force is transmitted to the distal humerus from the radius, which results in a shearing force across the capitellum in the coronal plane. Other mechanisms resulting in this injury include a direct blow, with the elbow flexed.

On physical examination, crepitus with elbow flexion and extension, and limited range of motion or impingement is often present. Pain is localized along the lateral aspect of the elbow. Examination of the elbow may be difficult because of global elbow pain from the fracture and soft tissue injury with swelling. In addition to examination of the elbow, a thorough evaluation of the wrist and shoulder is necessary to rule out associated injuries. Concomitant injuries may include radial head fractures, medial and lateral collateral ligament injuries, and elbow dislocation.

Classification

Bryan and Morrey [1] classified fractures of the capitellum into three patterns. Type I is a coronal shear fracture through the capitellum, resulting in a hemispheric fracture fragment, also called a Hahn-Steinthal fracture. This type is the most common. Type II involves a shell of articular cartilage with a thin layer of subchondral bone, and appears as though the capitellum has become "uncapped." This type is also known as a Kocher-Lorenz fracture. A type III fracture is comminuted, and often impacted. This type is associated more commonly with radial head fractures (Fig. 1). McKee and colleagues [4] described a fourth type, a shear fracture including the capitellum and extending medially into most of the trochlea (Fig. 2).

Recently, Ring and colleagues [6] proposed a new classification system for articular fractures of the distal humerus, consisting of five patterns of injury (Fig. 3). The investigators describe several variants of intra-articular fractures following higher-energy trauma to the elbow. Type 1 consists of a single articular fragment that includes the capitellum and lateral trochlea, which is similar to a Hahn-Steinthal fracture. Type 2 is a type 1 fracture with an associated lateral epicondyle fracture. Type 3 is a type 2 fracture with impaction of the metaphyseal bone in the posterolateral aspect of the lateral column. Type 4 is a type 3 fracture with a fracture of the posterior aspect of the trochlea. Type 5 is a type 4 fracture with fracture of the medial epicondyle.

Imaging studies

Fractures of the distal humerus may be difficult to assess, and may be easily missed on standard radiographs. It is essential to obtain true lateral and anterior-posterior views because obliquity of the lateral view may obscure visualization of the fracture. The posterior fat pad sign may be helpful in diagnosis of an intra-articular fracture. Because

E-mail address: evcheung@stanford.edu

0749-0712/07/$ - see front matter
doi:10.1016/j.hcl.2007.08.001

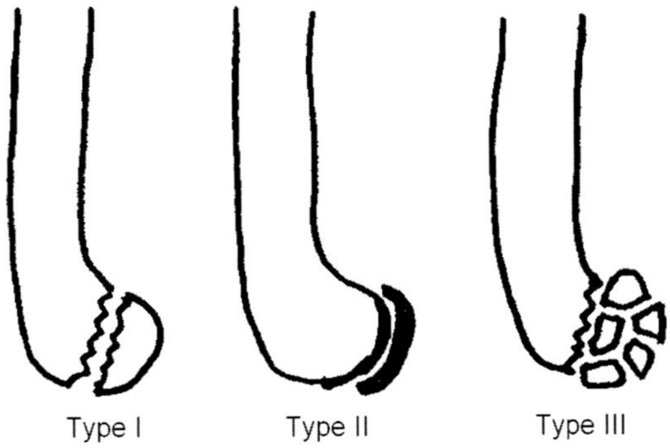

Fig. 1. Fractures of the capitellum. Type I, coronal shear fracture. Type II, articular shear fracture. Type III, comminuted fracture.

the fracture fragments include large cartilaginous components, radiographs often underestimate the size of the fragment. A "double-arc" sign has been noted on lateral radiographs when the capitellum fracture involves a large part of the trochlea (Fig. 4).

CT scans with axial, sagittal, coronal, and three-dimensional reconstructions may be necessary for the surgeon to understand the anatomy of the fracture for preoperative planning. These scans are especially useful when evaluating for concomitant injuries, such as a transcondylar or intercondylar distal humerus fracture, with a capitellar fracture component. On the CT scan, if the fracture extends into the medial epicondyle or if posterior involvement of the trochlea is indicated, the preferred surgical approach might be through an olecranon osteotomy. Concomitant capitellar fractures and radial head fractures may be missed on plain radiographs, but diagnosed on CT scan [10].

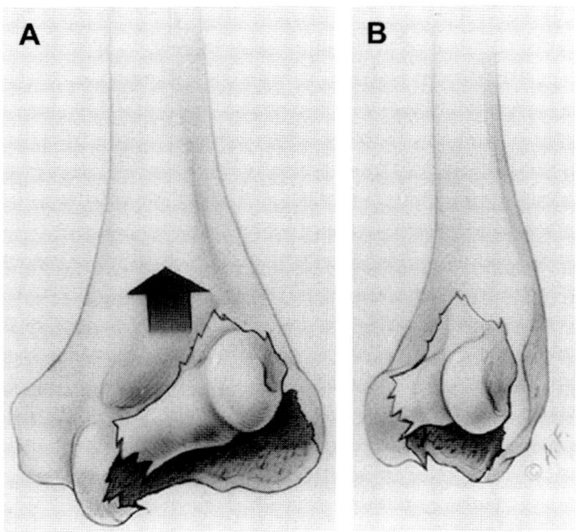

Fig. 2. Type IV capitellar fracture as described by McKee et al [4]. (*A*) Anterior view showing the fracture, which includes most of the anterior joint surface. The arrow represents direction of displacement of the fragment. (*B*) Oblique view showing the fracture line in the coronal plane. (*From* McKee MD, Jupiter J, Bamberger H. Coronal shear fractures of the distal end of the humerus. J Bone Joint Surg Am 1996;78:49–54; with permission.)

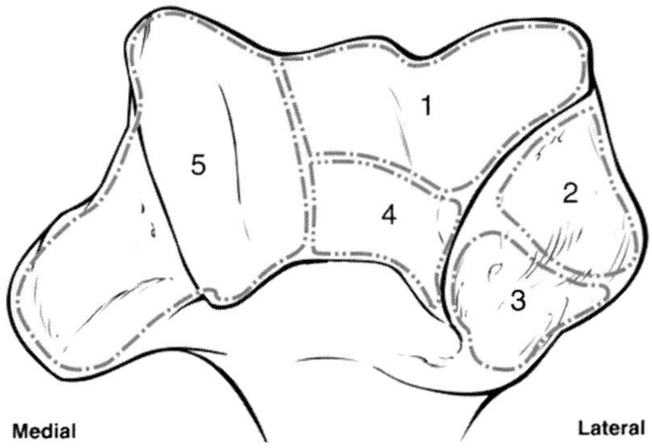

Fig. 3. Articular surface of the distal part of the humerus, demonstrating the locations of the five components of articular fractures. (*From* Ring D, Jupiter J, Gulotta L. Articular fractures of the distal part of the humerus. J Bone Joint Surg Am 2003;85:232–8; with permission.)

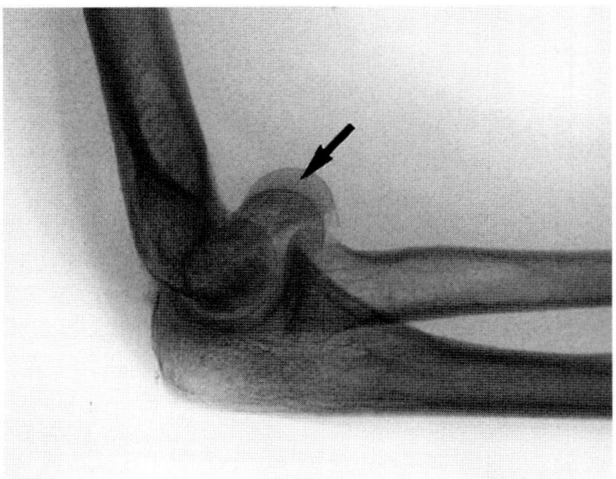

Fig. 4. Lateral radiograph of the elbow, showing the characteristic double-arc sign (*arrow*). One arc represents the subchondral bone of the capitellum, and the other, the lateral ridge of the trochlea. (*From* McKee MD, Jupiter J, Bamberger H. Coronal shear fractures of the distal end of the humerus. J Bone Joint Surg Am 1996;78:49–54; with permission.)

Treatment

Operative repair of capitellar fractures may be technically challenging. The surgeon must be prepared to perform an extensile operative exposure for realignment of small articular fragments. Implants must be countersunk beneath the articular surface. Open reduction internal fixation of displaced fractures of the capitellum is recommended to achieve healing of the fracture and to facilitate recovery of elbow motion. This fixation has been described using various methods, such as with variable pitch headless screws [3,4,7,11], plates [9], Kirschner wires, and bioabsorbable pins [12,13]. The benefit of variable pitch headless screws is that compression may be applied across the fracture. If anatomic and stable reduction of type II or type III fractures cannot be achieved because of the small size of the fragments, then excision of the fragments is recommended [14,15].

Surgical technique

Closed management is a reasonable treatment option when strict anatomic alignment of the fracture can be maintained. However, reduction maneuvers may be difficult to perform in swollen elbows, and even slight residual displacement of the fracture may result in significant loss of motion. Prolonged immobilization following closed reduction often leads to elbow stiffness. If comminution has occurred, the fracture fragments may act as loose bodies, and mechanically block elbow motion.

Hence, most investigators recommend operative treatment of capitellar fractures. Management of type I and type IV fractures is with operative fixation. Most type II and III fractures are treated with excision of the fragments. A lateral approach to the elbow is typically used when the medial extension of the fracture is limited. The skin incision is centered at the lateral epicondyle, extending proximally a few centimeters, and distally to the level of the radial head. Alternatively, a posterior longitudinal skin incision may be used, with a full-thickness skin flap created laterally. The benefit of a posterior skin incision is in its versatility; it also affords access laterally and medially, if needed (Fig. 5A, B).

The lateral column of the distal humerus is identified. Kaplan's interval is used between the extensor digitorum communis and the extensor carpi radialis longus, to preserve the lateral ulnar collateral ligament (LUCL) attachment site at the lateral epicondyle. If visualization is needed more distally, the LUCL may be released from the epicondyle, but care is taken to reattach it at the end of the procedure. Alternatively, Kocher's interval between the extensor carpi ulnaris and the anconeus may be used to obtain better visualization posteriorly than with Kaplan's interval. Care is taken to repair the LUCL at the end of the procedure. If the epicondyle is fractured, the fragment is reflected distally and repaired after fixation of the articular fragments. The common extensors are elevated anteriorly off the supracondylar ridge as a full-thickness sleeve, and the anterior capsule is elevated in continuity with this sleeve of tissue to provide ample visualization of the anterior elbow joint. A blunt Hohmann retractor is placed beneath the anterior capsule around to the medial aspect of the humerus.

The exposure is enhanced by elevating the lateral triceps from the humerus and olecranon, if necessary, which permits the elbow to be hinged open slightly and provides exposure of the anterior and posterior articular surfaces of the distal humerus. The common extensors are repaired back either to a cuff of tissue left on the humerus or to the lateral triceps fascia at the end of the case.

A posterior approach with an olecranon osteotomy provides better visualization of the distal humeral articular surface when the medial extension of the fracture fragments is significant, and it may be necessary for such cases. A posterior skin incision is used. Full-thickness skin flaps are created medially and laterally. The ulnar nerve is mobilized and transposed anteriorly into a subcutaneous pocket. An apex distal chevron osteotomy is created with an oscillating saw at the midlevel of the olecranon. The olecranon fragment and triceps are then reflected proximally. The osteotomy may be repaired with a figure-of-eight tension band construct using stainless-steel wire in combination with either two parallel Kirschner wires or a 6.5- or 7.5-mm cannulated screw; alternatively, plate fixation may be used.

The capitellar fracture fragments are identified and may be reduced through Kaplan's interval, or through Kocher's approach, which exposes the posterior column. The fracture is reduced with extension, supination, and a varus force. The elbow is then flexed, once the fragment is slid distally to be captured by the radial head. The reduction maneuver may be difficult because of the lack of soft tissue attachments to the articular fragments. The fragment is provisionally fixed

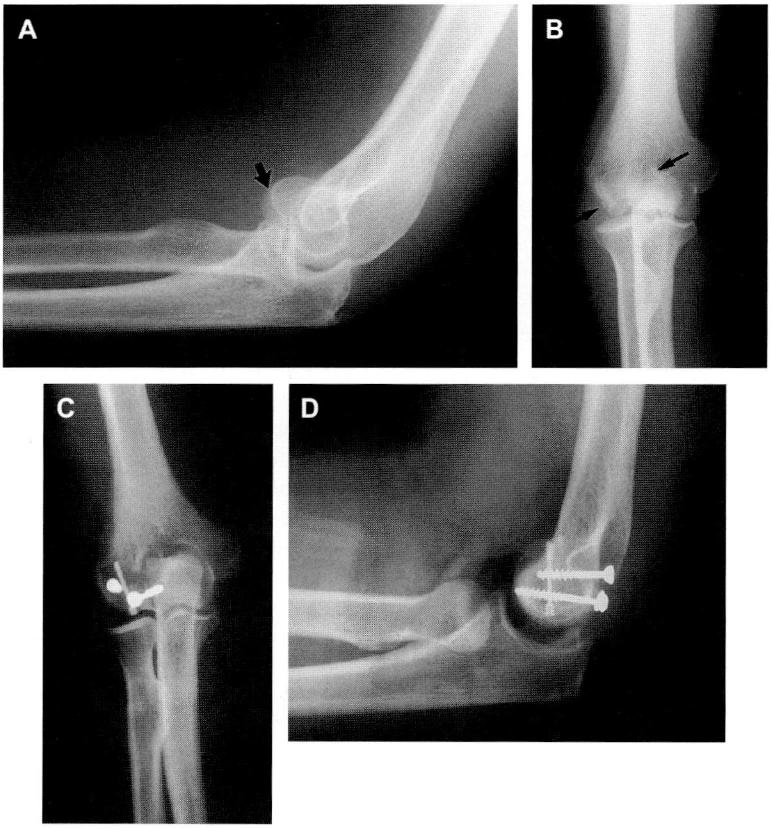

Fig. 5. (*A* and *B*) Preoperative anteroposterior and lateral radiographs of a type IV capitellar fracture. (*A*) The arrow represents the "so-called" double-arc sign. (*B*) The arrows demonstrate the lateral and medial borders of the fracture. (*C* and *D*) Postoperative anteroposterior and lateral radiographs after open reduction internal fixation with Herbert screw and 4.0-mm partially threaded cannulated screws. (*From* McKee MD, Jupiter J, Bamberger H. Coronal shear fractures of the distal end of the humerus. J Bone Joint Surg Am 1996;78:49–54; with permission.)

with smooth Kirschner wires. Definitive fixation of the fracture fragments is achieved with countersunk headless screws placed perpendicular to the fracture line, from anterior to posterior, or from posterior to anterior if possible, in divergent orientation [2,4,7,16]. Ideally, two screws are used for rotational stability.

Anatomic alignment may not possible because of impaction of the posterior trochlea or the posterior aspect of the lateral column. The surgeon should recognize that the inferior aspect of the capitellum is often comminuted and should not be used as a reference for final reduction. Autogenous cancellous bone graft from the iliac crest or olecranon may be packed into such posterior defects.

In type III fractures with extensive comminution, or when the posterolateral column is fractured, it may be technically challenging to place screws. The lateral epicondyle with the attached LUCL can be reflected distally to afford adequate exposure. Fixation using absorbable pins has been described [2]. A stable bony column for reattachment of the articular fragments must be identified. If fragments are too small to accept fixation with bioabsorbable pins or Kirschner wires, they may be removed. A precontoured lateral column plate may be secured onto the lateral column to augment fixation. A maxillofacial inverted Y-plate has also been used for fixation of capitellar fractures, with good to excellent results [9].

Elbow range of motion is assessed to ensure no impingement or crepitus after fixation. The forearm is also rotated to ensure that the radial head articulates congruently with the capitellum in full pronation and supination. Intraoperative fluoroscopy is routinely used. The elbow is placed into a splint at 90° of flexion.

Postoperative rehabilitation

The splint is removed in approximately 1 week, and the patient is encouraged to do gentle active range of motion exercises without the aid of a physical therapist. When extensive intra-articular comminution has occurred and the stability of the internal fixation is uncertain, the elbow may need to be immobilized for a longer period of time. Formal physical therapy for passive range of motion and strengthening is not started until bony healing is evident, at about 6 to 8 weeks postoperatively. Patients are given oral indomethacin (25 mg, three times daily), for 4 weeks to minimize the possibility of heterotopic ossification, if they do not have a history of peptic ulcer disease. However, the use of indomethacin has not been universally reported, and its use is surgeon-dependent.

Results

Gratham and colleagues [17] reported the results of 29 capitellar fractures that included 19 type I, 2 type II, and 8 type III fractures. They concluded that type I fractures should be treated with open reduction internal fixation (ORIF) if closed reduction is unsuccessful in young, healthy patients. For elderly patients who have type I fractures, excision of the fragment may be a reasonable option. For type II and type III fractures, good results were reported with excision of the fragments.

Recently, Mighell and colleagues [2] reported on their series of 16 patients who had operative fixation of capitellar fractures using a lateral approach, and fixation with either headless screws or bioabsorbable pins, and posterolateral column plates when indicated. This series included eight type I, two type III, and six type IV capitellar fractures, with a mean follow-up of 13 months. According to the Broberg-Morrey scale [18], 11 fractures had excellent results and 5 had good results. Fracture union was achieved in all cases. The average arc of motion was 124°, and the average flexion contracture was 13°. The four complications consisted of two patients who had radiographic evidence of mild radiocapitellar arthrosis and two patients who had grade 1 heterotopic ossification.

Ring and colleagues [6] reported on 21 patients who had operative fixation of capitellar fractures using buried implants, and either a lateral or a posterior approach using an olecranon osteotomy (for type 5 fractures). Average follow-up was 40 months. According to the Mayo Elbow Performance Score (MEPS), 4 patients had excellent results, 12 had good results, and 5 had fair results. Ten of the 21 patients required a second operation: 6 for release of elbow contracture, 2 for treatment of ulnar neuropathy, 1 for removal of symptomatic hardware, and 1 for early loss of fixation of the capitellum. The release of elbow contractures improved an average of 42° of motion. When multiple articular fragments were impacted, postoperative immobilization was extended to several weeks, based on the tenet that a healed, stable, but stiff, elbow can later be treated by capsular releases to improve mobility. No cases of osteonecrosis were reported, despite the separation of the fracture fragments from metaphyseal bone and from soft tissue attachments.

Although earlier reports indicated no cases of osteonecrosis or collapse in the region of the fracture, these have been documented with longer follow-up [3]. In addition, patients who have isolated noncomminuted fractures have better results than those with more complex fractures. Dubberley and colleagues [3] reported on the largest series of patients with open reduction internal fixation of these fractures. The series consisted of 28 patients with mean follow-up of 56 months. The average MEPS score was 91, and the average range of motion was 19° to 138°. Twelve of the 28 patients required a re-operation. Seven patients required capsulectomy and hardware removal for loss of motion. One patient had nonunion, treated by iliac crest bone grafting and placement of an external fixator. Two comminuted fractures did not unite and were converted to total elbow arthroplasties. One had nonunion of the olecranon osteotomy, and another had a painful elbow treated with hardware removal. Nine patients had posttraumatic arthritis classified according to the system of Broberg and Morrey [18], and three had osteonecrosis of the capitellum or trochlea. The use of maxillofacial Y-shaped plates for fixation of capitellar fractures has also been described with good to excellent results [9].

Articular cartilage injuries of the posterolateral capitellum caused by shearing have also been found intraoperatively at the time of operative treatment for radial head fractures, as described by Caputo and colleagues [10]. At that time, an unexpected shear fracture of the capitellar articular cartilage was wedged into the radial head fracture, blocking reduction. Of the 10 patients in their cohort, none of the injuries were identified on preoperative imaging. The capitellar fragments were too small to support stable internal fixation and were therefore excised, and the defect in the capitellum was debrided of loose edges in all cases. No sequelae were identified on short-term follow-up.

If anatomic and stable reduction of type II fractures cannot be achieved, excision of the fragments is a possible treatment option. Arthroscopic excision of type II capitellar fractures in two cases was reported by Feldman [15]. In experienced hands, arthroscopic excision of type II fractures may be a safe, effective technique that allows intra-articular inspection of the elbow for occult injuries.

Summary

Fractures of the capitellum are rare, but can lead to significant disability because of limitation of elbow motion and arthrosis. Internal fixation by various methods has been described, with good results overall. Restoring the anatomy of the radiohumeral articulation with rigid fixation is important for restoring early mobility to the elbow.

References

[1] Bryan R, Morrey B. Fractures of the distal humerus. In: Morrey B, editor. The elbow and its disorders. Philadelphia: WB Saunders; 1985. p. 325–33.

[2] Mighell MA, Harkins D, Klein D, et al. Technique for internal fixation of capitellum and lateral trochlea fractures. J Orthop Trauma 2006;20:699–704.

[3] Dubberley JH, Faber KJ, Macdermid JC, et al. Outcome after open reduction and internal fixation of capitellar and trochlear fractures. J Bone Joint Surg 2006;88:46–54.

[4] McKee MD, Jupiter J, Bamberger H. Coronal shear fractures of the distal end of the humerus. J Bone Joint Surg 1996;78:49–54.

[5] Pogliacomi F, Concari G, Vaienti E. Hahn-Steinthal fracture: report of two cases. Acta Biomed 2005;76: 178–84.

[6] Ring D, Jupiter J, Gulotta L. Articular fractures of the distal part of the humerus. J Bone Joint Surg 2003;85:232–8.

[7] Sano S, Rokkaku T, Saito S, et al. Herbert screw fixation of capitellar fractures. J Shoulder Elbow Surg 2005;14:307–11.

[8] Poynton AR, Kelly IP, O'Rourke SK. Fractures of the capitellum–a comparison of two fixation methods. Injury 1998;29:341–3.

[9] Clough TM, Jago ER, Sidhu DP, et al. Fractures of the capitellum: a new method of fixation using a maxillofacial plate. Clin Orthop Relat Res 2001;232–6.

[10] Caputo AE, Burton KJ, Cohen MS, et al. Articular cartilage injuries of the capitellum interposed in radial head fractures: a report of ten cases. J Shoulder Elbow Surg 2006;15:716–20.

[11] Liberman N, Katz T, Howard CB, et al. Fixation of capitellar fractures with the Herbert screw. Arch Orthop Trauma Surg 1991;110:155–7.

[12] Bilic R, Kolundzic R, Anticevic D. Absorbable implants in surgical correction of a capitellar malunion in an 11-year-old: a case report. J Orthop Trauma 2006;20:66–9.

[13] Hirvensalo E, Bostman O, Partio E, et al. Fracture of the humeral capitellum fixed with absorbable polyglycolide pins. 1-year follow-up of 8 adults. Acta Orthop Scand 1993;64:85–6.

[14] Alvarez E, Patel MR, Nimberg G, et al. Fracture of the capitulum humeri. In, vol 57; 1975. p. 1093–96.

[15] Feldman MD. Arthroscopic excision of type II capitellar fractures. Arthroscopy 1997;13:743–8.

[16] Pearce MS, Gallannaugh SC. Mason type II radial head fractures fixed with Herbert bone screws. J R Soc Med 1996;89:340P–4P.

[17] Gratham S, Norris T, Bush D. Isolated fracture of the humeral capitellum. Clin Orthop Relat Res 1981;161:262–9.

[18] Broberg MA, Morrey BF. Results of treatment of fracture-dislocations of the elbow. Clin Orthop Relat Res 1987;216:109–19.

ELSEVIER SAUNDERS

Hand Clin 23 (2007) 487–490

HAND CLINICS

Index

Note: Page numbers of article titles are in **boldface** type.

doi:10.1016/S0749-0712(07)00103-5

hand.theclinics.com

T

U

United States Postal Service

Statement of Ownership, Management, and Circulation
(All Periodicals Publications Except Requestor Publications)

1. Publication Title	2. Publication Number	3. Filing Date
Hand Clinics	0 0 0 - 7 0 9	9/14/07
4. Issue Frequency: Feb, May, Aug, Nov	5. Number of Issues Published Annually: 4	6. Annual Subscription Price: $237.00

7. Complete Mailing Address of Known Office of Publication (*Not printer*) (*Street, city, county, state, and ZIP+4*)

Elsevier Inc.
360 Park Avenue South
New York, NY 10010-1710

Contact Person: Stephen Bushing
Telephone (Include area code): 215-239-3688

8. Complete Mailing Address of Headquarters or General Business Office of Publisher (*Not printer*)

Elsevier Inc., 360 Park Avenue South, New York, NY 10010-1710

9. Full Names and Complete Mailing Addresses of Publisher, Editor, and Managing Editor (*Do not leave blank*)

Publisher (*Name and complete mailing address*)

John Schrefer , Elsevier, Inc., 1600 John F. Kennedy Blvd. Suite 1800, Philadelphia, PA 19103-2899

Editor (*Name and complete mailing address*)

Deb Dellapena, Elsevier, Inc., 1600 John F. Kennedy Blvd. Suite 1800, Philadelphia, PA 19103-2899

Managing Editor (*Name and complete mailing address*)

Catherine Bewick, Elsevier, Inc., 1600 John F. Kennedy Blvd. Suite 1800, Philadelphia, PA 19103-2899

10. Owner (*Do not leave blank. If the publication is owned by a corporation, give the name and address of the corporation immediately followed by the names and addresses of all stockholders owning or holding 1 percent or more of the total amount of stock. If not owned by a corporation, give the names and addresses of the individual owners. If owned by a partnership or other unincorporated firm, give its name and address as well as those of each individual owner. If the publication is published by a nonprofit organization, give its name and address.*)

Full Name	Complete Mailing Address
Wholly owned subsidiary of	4520 East-West Highway
Reed/Elsevier, US holdings	Bethesda, MD 20814

11. Known Bondholders, Mortgagees, and Other Security Holders Owning or Holding 1 Percent or More of Total Amount of Bonds, Mortgages, or Other Securities. If none, check box → None

Full Name	Complete Mailing Address
N/A	

12. Tax Status (*For completion by nonprofit organizations authorized to mail at nonprofit rates*) (*Check one*)
The purpose, function, and nonprofit status of this organization and the exempt status for federal income tax purposes:
Has Not Changed During Preceding 12 Months
Has Changed During Preceding 12 Months (*Publisher must submit explanation of change with this statement*)

PS Form 3526, September 2006 (Page 1 of 3 (Instructions Page 3)) PSN 7530-01-000-9931 **PRIVACY NOTICE**: See our Privacy policy in www.usps.com

13. Publication Title: Hand Clinics
14. Issue Date for Circulation Data Below: May 2007

15. Extent and Nature of Circulation			Average No. Copies Each Issue During Preceding 12 Months	No. Copies of Single Issue Published Nearest to Filing Date
a. Total Number of Copies (*Net press run*)			2600	2600
b. Paid Circulation (By Mail and Outside the Mail)	(1)	Mailed Outside-County Paid Subscriptions Stated on PS Form 3541. (*Include paid distribution above nominal rate, advertiser's proof copies, and exchange copies*)	1369	1283
	(2)	Mailed In-County Paid Subscriptions Stated on PS Form 3541 (*Include paid distribution above nominal rate, advertiser's proof copies, and exchange copies*)		
	(3)	Paid Distribution Outside the Mails Including Sales Through Dealers and Carriers, Street Vendors, Counter Sales, and Other Paid Distribution Outside USPS®	471	439
	(4)	Paid Distribution by Other Classes Mailed Through the USPS (e.g. First-Class Mail®)		
c. Total Paid Distribution (*Sum of 15b (1), (2), (3), and (4)*) ►			1840	1722
d. Free or Nominal Rate Distribution (By Mail and Outside the Mail)	(1)	Free or Nominal Rate Outside-County Copies Included on PS Form 3541	117	82
	(2)	Free or Nominal Rate In-County Copies Included on PS Form 3541		
	(3)	Free or Nominal Rate Copies Mailed at Other Classes Mailed Through the USPS (e.g. First-Class Mail)		
	(4)	Free or Nominal Rate Distribution Outside the Mail (Carriers or other means)		
e. Total Free or Nominal Rate Distribution (Sum of 15d (1), (2), (3) and (4)			117	82
f. Total Distribution (Sum of 15c and 15e) ►			1957	1804
g. Copies not Distributed (See instructions to publishers #4 (page #3)) ►			643	796
h. Total (Sum of 15f and g)			2600	2600
i. Percent Paid (15c divided by 15f times 100) ►			94.02%	95.45%

16. Publication of Statement of Ownership

If the publication is a general publication, publication of this statement is required. Will be printed in the **November 2007** issue of this publication. Publication not required

17. Signature and Title of Editor, Publisher, Business Manager, or Owner

Jean Fanucci – Executive Director of Subscription Services — Date: September 14, 2007

I certify that all information furnished on this form is true and complete. I understand that anyone who furnishes false or misleading information on this form or who omits material or information requested on the form may be subject to criminal sanctions (including fines and imprisonment) and/or civil sanctions (including civil penalties).

PS Form 3526, September 2006 (Page 2 of 3)